Nursing Pathways
for
Patient Safety

National Council of State Boards of Nursing (NCSBN)
Expert Panel on Practice Breakdown

NCSBN
National Council of State Boards of Nursing

Patricia E. Benner, PhD, RN, FAAN, *Editor/Contributor*
Kathy Malloch, PhD, MBA, RN, FAAN, *Editor/Contributor*
Vickie Sheets, JD, RN, CAE, *Editor/Contributor*

Karla Bitz, PhD, RN, *Contributor*
Kathy A. Scott, PhD, CHE, RN, *Contributor*
Lisa Emrich, MSN, RN, *Contributor*
Mary Beth Thomas, MSN, PhD(c), RN, *Contributor*
Kathryn Schwed, JD, *Contributor*
Vicki Goettsche, BSN, MBA, RN, *Contributor*
Linda Patterson, BSN, RN, *Contributor*
Karen Bowen, MS, RN, *Contributor*
Kevin Kenward, PhD, *Contributor*

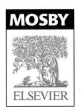

MOSBY

ELSEVIER

MOSBY
ELSEVIER

3251 Riverport Lane
St. Louis, Missouri 63043

Nursing Pathways for Patient Safety   ISBN: 978-0-323-06517-7

Notice

Library of Congress Cataloging-in-Publication Data

National Council of State Boards of Nursing (U.S.). Expert Panel on Practice Breakdown.
  Nursing pathways for patient safety / National Council of State Boards of Nursing (NCSBN), Expert Panel on Practice Breakdown ; Patricia E. Benner, Kathy Malloch, Vickie Sheets, editors; Karla Bitz ... [et al.]. – 1st ed.
     p. ; cm.
  Includes bibliographical references and index.
  ISBN 978-0-323-06517-7 (pbk. : alk. paper)
  1. Nursing errors. 2. Nursing–Practice. I. Benner, Patricia E. II. Malloch, Kathy. III. Sheets, Vickie IV. Title.
  [DNLM: 1. Nursing Care–Practice Guideline. 2. Medical Errors–prevention & control–Practice Guideline. WY 100 N2726n 2010]
  RT85.6.N38 2010
  610.73068–dc22

2009022215

Senior Editor: Lee Henderson
Senior Developmental Editor: Rae Robertson
Publishing Services Manager: Gayle May
Project Manager: Tracey Schriefer
Designer: Kimberly Denando

Printed in the United States of America
Last digit is the print number: 9 8 7 6 5 4

ABOUT THE EDITOR/CONTRIBUTOR TEAM

Patricia E. Benner, *PhD, RN, FAAN,* is Consultant to the NCSBN Expert Panel on Practice Breakdown and is Professor of Nursing, University of California, San Francisco. Dr. Benner has served as Consultant to the Panel since its inception in 1999.

Kathy Malloch, *PhD, MBA, RN, FAAN,* is Chairperson of the NCSBN Expert Panel on Practice Breakdown. She is also President of Malloch & Associates, Director of the Master's In Healthcare Innovation Program at Arizona State University, and President of the Arizona State Board of Nursing. Dr. Malloch served as a member of the Panel from 1999 to 2001 and has served as Chairperson of the Panel since 2001.

Vickie Sheets, *JD, RN, CAE,* serves as Staff Member of the NCSBN Expert Panel on Practice Breakdown and is the Director of Practice and Regulation, NCSBN. Ms. Sheets has worked with the Panel since its inception.

ABOUT THE CONTRIBUTORS

Karla Bitz, *PhD, RN,* is a member of the NCSBN Expert Panel on Practice Breakdown and Associate Director of the North Dakota Board of Nursing. Dr. Bitz's tenure on the Panel was from 2001 to 2006.

Kathy A. Scott, *PhD, CHE, RN,* is Consultant to the NCSBN Expert Panel on Practice Breakdown and Vice-President of Clinical Services, Banner Health, Arizona Region. Dr. Scott's consultancy with the Panel was from 2002 to 2006.

Lisa Emrich, *MSN, RN,* is a member of the NCSBN Expert Panel on Practice Breakdown and Manager of the Education, Practice and Alternative Programs Unit, Ohio Board of Nursing. Ms. Emrich served on the Panel from 2002 to 2006.

Mary Beth Thomas, *MSN, PhD(c), RN,* is a member of the NCSBN Expert Panel on Practice Breakdown and Director of Nursing of the Texas Board of Nurse Examiners. Ms. Thomas served on the Panel from 2004 to 2006.

Kathryn Schwed, *JD,* is a member of the NCSBN Expert Panel on Practice Breakdown and attorney for the New Jersey State Board of Nursing. Ms. Schwed was a member of the Panel from 1999 to 2006.

Vicki Goettsche, *BSN, MBA, RN,* is a member of the NCSBN Expert Panel on Practice Breakdown and Associate Director of the Idaho State Board of Registered Nursing. Ms. Goettsche was a member of the Panel from 2002 to 2006.

Linda Patterson, *BSN, RN,* is a member of the NCSBN Expert Panel on Practice Breakdown and a Healthcare Investigator for the Washington State Nursing Care Quality Assurance Commission. Ms. Patterson served on the Panel from 2002 to 2006.

Karen Bowen, *MS, RN,* is a member of the NCSBN Expert Panel on Practice Breakdown and is Nursing Practice Consultant for the Nebraska Board of Nursing. Ms. Bowen served on the Panel from 2004 to 2006.

Kevin Kenward, *PhD,* serves as Staff Member of the NCSBN Expert Panel on Practice Breakdown and is Director of Research for the NCSBN. Dr. Kenward has worked with the Panel since January 2005.

I have always said that the most significant work of the National Council of State Boards of Nursing, Inc. (NCSBN®) starts with a good question. Inevitably, the strategic initiatives of the NCSBN that have the greatest impact in the public protection arena begin with a simple but profound question. The question for this book emerged from a discussion of the discipline function at state boards of nursing. All state boards of nursing in their public protection mandate must ensure that nurses are safe and competent to practice at the time of initial licensure and throughout their entire career in order to protect the consumer. When evidence of substandard nursing practice demonstrates a clear violation of state law or the Nurse Practice Act, boards of nursing are mandated to take action through administrative procedures that result in discipline of the nurse. The process is reactive; the challenge exists in making it a more proactive.

How can state boards of nursing be proactive and prevent unsafe practice? If this question is answered, patient safety would be improved. Additionally, prevention of unsafe practice decreases the need for the disciplinary administrative process, which typically accounts for the largest portion of a board of nursing's annual budget.

So what do we know about nursing practice that results in disciplinary action? We certainly know a fair amount about the disciplinary process, since this is an integral function of any health care licensing board. We have data on the types of disciplinary actions taken and a general idea of what brings nursing practice to the attention of the state board of nursing. What we had not studied was the phenomenon of what happens when nursing practice breaks down from both a system and an individual point of view.

The NCSBN is an organization founded by state boards of nursing to decrease government burdens. It does this by providing an organization through which boards of nursing act on matters of common interest and concern affecting the public health, safety, and welfare. A mainstay of this organization is the creation of committees composed of board of nursing staff as well as nurses and other experts appointed to serve the boards.

These committees convene to research regulatory issues, develop regulatory models, create position papers, and provide the analysis that forms the foundation for evidenced-based regulatory decisions.

Since 2002 the mission of the NCSBN has been rooted in the concept of regulatory excellence and its advancement. State boards of nursing recognize that good solid data are needed to create effective public policy and further the evolution of nursing practice regulation.

In 2002 the Practice Breakdown Research Advisory Panel was created to develop a collection instrument that would extract data from disciplinary cases. The data collected would record the incident, the individual nurse involved, and the system in which the incident occurred. The NCSBN invited experts to participate in this process and was honored to have Dr. Patricia Benner, Dr. Kathy Scott, and Dr. Marie Farrell as participants along with members from state boards of nursing and NCSBN staff. The work of the Advisory Panel clearly aligned with the strategic direction of the organization regarding regulatory excellence.

Taxonomy of Error, Root Cause Analysis, and Practice Responsibility (TERCAP®) was launched in February 2007 as a secure and comprehensive online intake instrument designed for nursing boards to use prospectively in cases involving practice breakdown. Study questions from this book will be used to analyze the aggregate data that nursing boards will report to the NCSBN.

This book and the work it represents have had the complete support of the Board of Directors and NCSBN staff throughout the entire process. As the executive director of the NCSBN, I knew from the beginning that the potential of this project would have a dramatic impact on patient safety in this country. The data collected from the use of the TERCAP instrument and resulting analysis will provide critical patient safety improvement information, the likes of which have not been seen in other studies.

George Bernard Shaw said, "No question is so difficult to answer as that to which the answer is obvious." This book answers the question, and in the future TERCAP will continue to uncover data that will contribute to the improvement of nursing practices and the protection of the public.

Kathy Apple, MS, RN, CAE
Chief Executive Officer
National Council of State Boards of Nursing

The goal of this work is to better understand and articulate the role of nurses, health care institutions, working conditions, and education on patient safety. Nurses are the last possible point of preventing errors in health care because they are the ones to monitor patients and deliver most therapies. Some areas of patient safety receive more emphasis, such as medication error and surgical mishaps, yet focus on these two areas of patient safety cause the public to overlook large areas of patient safety, such as lack of prevention of hazards of immobility and hospitalization, and errors related to patient vulnerabilities, such as cognitive impairment, allergies, and physical limitations. The state boards of nursing identified a need for broadening the focus on patient safety and on the role of nurses in patient safety.

This is a landmark work of the NCSBN to communicate recent changes in investigatory tools, including a taxonomy of standards of nursing practice that are at the frontline of patient safety work. The impetus for this work was to delineate the very general and broad category of professional nursing actions and judgments into distinct functions, goals, and notions of good internal to nursing practice. All professional nursing actions might be considered to be based on good judgment and the standards of good nursing practice, but distinct aspects of frontline nursing aims, such as preventing the hazards of immobility and safety risks due to hospitalization, are attended to primarily by nurses. Even the safety measures instituted for other professional workers are monitored and maintained by nurses. The impetus for this work was also to respond to the Institute of Medicine reports on patient safety (Kohn, L.T., Corrigan, J.M., & Donaldson, M.S., 2000) by developing more standardized investigatory categories that incorporate systems issues, including environmental issues, team functioning, staffing, a nurse's work patterns, as well as the usual focus on the professional nurse's narrative account of the reported incident and an assessment of responsibility and accountability in a particular incident of practice breakdown. The goal is to develop a national database of nursing errors/practice breakdown reported to state boards of nursing in order to improve the prevention of errors, and increase the research base for disciplinary and educational strategies to improve patient safety on the part of nurses. A secondary goal is to make the TERCAP tool of describing nursing practice breakdown available to hospitals and other health care institutions.

We believe that this work will help nurses and student nurses improve their practice and better understand the kinds of practice breakdown incidents that might be reported to the state boards of nursing. The focus of the book is on the broad dimensions of patient safety work that have always been central to the nursing role, since nurses are at the sharp end of practice (Kohn et al., 2000) and the patient's last line of defense for the prevention of errors. These broad categories will be explicated and illustrated throughout the book as follows: (1) *Safe Medication Administration*: The nurse administers the right dose of the right medication via the right route to the right patient at the right time for the right reason. (2) *Documentation*: Nursing documentation provides relevant information about the patient and the measures implemented in response to their needs. (3) *Attentiveness/Surveillance*: The nurse monitors what is happening with the patient and staff. The nurse observes the patient's clinical condition. If the nurse has not observed a patient, then he/she cannot identify changes if they have occurred and/or make knowledgeable discernments and decisions about the patient's condition or care. (4) *Clinical Reasoning*: Nurses interpret patients' signs, symptoms, and responses to therapies. Nurses evaluate the relevance of changes in patients' signs and symptoms and ensure that patient care providers are notified and that patient care is adjusted appropriately. (5) *Prevention*: The nurse follows usual and customary measures to prevent risks, hazards, or complications due to illness or hospitalization. These include taking precautions to prevent falls and preventing the hazards of immobility, contractures, or stasis pneumonia, and more. (6) *Intervention*: The nurse properly executes nursing interventions. (7) *Interpretation of Authorized Provider Orders*: The nurse interprets authorized provider orders. (8) *Professional Responsibility/Patient Advocacy*: The nurse demonstrates professional responsibility and understands the nature of the nurse-patient relationship. Advocacy refers to the expectations that nurses act responsibly in protecting patient/family vulnerabilities and in advocating to see that patient needs/concerns are addressed.

At the heart of the work is the view that, ultimately, a narrow focus on discrete "errors" will not improve patient safety systems and nurse practice environments. In most cases it is a combination of practice styles, environments, teamwork, and structural systems that contribute to practice breakdown, a term used throughout this book instead of "mistakes" or the identification of single end points in error events.

Health care institutions are complex institutions that require professional knowledge workers who work in teams in legally bounded areas of responsibility for patient care (Sullivan, 2004; Benner & Sullivan, 2005). Rules, procedures, policies, and systems approaches to error prevention are essential but not sufficient for the daily practice of professionals who assume ethical and fiduciary responsibility for the prevention of harm, safe health care delivery, and facilitation of beneficial care toward the care and recovery of patients.

The work of nursing regulation is challenged, contentious, and resisted. Yet the need for an effective oversight process for patient safety and nurse competence has never been greater. The challenges of supply, demand, allocation of funding, role evolution, technology, and computerization advances and unprecedented consumerism have made the work of the NCSBN Practice Breakdown Advisory Panel (PBAP) not only an imperative for patient care quality but also a labor of love for panel members.

We created this book with the following goals in mind:
1. To transform the management of discipline using an evidence-based approach.
2. To provide objective and measurable insight into the practice of nursing as related to breakdown.
3. To provide a data collection instrument for nurse regulators, practitioners, and educators to assess and report consistently and objectively practice breakdown.

4. To begin to build a national repository of data that would better inform nursing practice and the solutions to improved and safer practice
5. To develop a taxonomy of nursing errors to better understand and articulate the nurse's role in patient safety.
6. To inform nurses, nurse educators and nursing students, patient safety managers, and policy makers about the types of errors reported to state boards of nursing and the disciplinary investigation processes related to those errors.

Creating this work has evolved much like an action research project—that is, as each phase was completed, new information became available and the next phase was launched. The PBAP began with the need to provide better informed discipline-specific decisions at the state level and ultimately produced a highly valid and reliable data collection instrument, the Taxonomy of Error, Root Cause Analysis, and Practice Responsibility (TERCAP®). This instrument is now available in electronic format to all boards of nursing in the United States and NCSBN territories. The term "root cause" is used in the title because the categories from a full root cause of analysis were used in the design of the instrument. The authors are clear that a survey including the categories usually covered in a root cause analysis is not the same, nor is a survey a replacement for the more lengthy local process of conducting an institutional root cause analysis. But as a survey instrument, used within a particular institution, the categories on the survey can be used for a statistical survey and compared to actual full-scale root cause analyses (Bagian, Gosbee, Lee, et al., 2002; Rex, Turnbull, Allen, et al., 2000; Chassin & Becher, 2002).

This book is organized to present the TERCAP and begins with an introduction to the years of work that informed its current format and content. Each of the TERCAP practice breakdown chapters is discussed in detail with definitions, explanations, and case examples. The book shows the ways in which the major elements of a framework evolved from a study of cases, and it ends with a brief summary of accomplishments and the panel's vision of the next steps needed to ensure a sound way forward to prevent practice breakdown in the health care workplace.

Kathy Malloch
Chairperson
NCSBN Expert Panel on Practice Breakdown

References

Bagian, J. P., Gosbee, J., & Lee, C. Z., et al. (2002). The Veterans Affairs root cause analysis system in action. *Joint Commission Journal on Quality Improvement, 28,* 531-545.

Benner, P., & Sullivan, W. (2005). Challenges to professionalism: work integrity and the call to renew and strengthen the social contract of the professions. *American Journal of Critical Care, 14*(1), 78-80, 84.

Chassin, M. R., & Becher E. C. (2002). The wrong patient. *Annals of Internal Medicine, 136,* 826-833.

Kohn, L. T., Corrigan, J. M., & Donaldson, M. S. (2000). To err is human: Building a safer health system. In: *Committee on Quality of Health Care in America.* Washington, DC: National Academy Press.

Rex, J. H., Turnbull, J. E., Allen S. J., et al. (2000). Systematic root cause analysis of adverse drug events in a tertiary referral hospital. *Joint Commission Journal on Quality Improvement, 26,* 563-575.

Sullivan, W. (2004). *Work and integrity: The crisis and promise of professionalism in America* (2nd ed.). San Francisco: Jossey-Bass.

ACKNOWLEDGMENTS

The editors would like to extend special thanks to the following people:

Angela Diaz-Kay is Director of Information Technology, NCSBN, and provided IT consultation from 1999 to 2005.

Marie P. Farrell, *EdD, MPH, RN, FAAN* is Consultant to the NCSBN Expert Panel on Practice Breakdown and Professor, Human and Organizational Development, Fielding Graduate University, Santa Barbara, California, and former European Advisor and Program Manager for Nursing, Midwifery, and Social Work, European Regional Office, World Health Organization, Copenhagen, Denmark. Dr. Farrell joined the Panel in June 2005.

Austin Garfield is an Information Technology Consultant and served as Temporary Consultant to the NCSBN from 2002 to 2004.

Angela Johnston served as Information Technology Consultant to the NCSBN from 2004 to 2006.

Dwane Jamison, *BA,* served as a member of the NCSBN Expert Panel from 1999 to 2004.

Patricia Uris, *PhD, RN,* served as First Chairperson of the Expert Panel from 1999 to 2001.

The editors and contributors also thank the hundreds of people who contributed to the research and other efforts needed to complete this book. Specifically, thanks are extended to the 16 boards of nursing in the United States and their staff for their help throughout the years of this project. These include the member boards in the states of: Arizona, Idaho, Iowa, New Jersey, North Dakota, Ohio, Texas, and Washington.

The editors and contributors are grateful to the staff members of the NCSBN for their diligence, efficiency, and ongoing competence in supporting the work of the project and its final products. Acknowledged are the following: Joey Ridenour, MN, RN, President of the NCSBN, who, in 1999, with Eloise Cathchart, MN, RN, former NCSBN Executive Director, established the Practice Breakdown Task Force. Also acknowledged is Donna Dorsey, MSN, RN, FAAN, Executive Director of the Maryland Board of Nursing from 2002 to 2006 and President of the NCSBN. Their foresight and wisdom were critical in conceptualizing the need for this work and for moving this need from idea to reality.

Sincere thanks are extended to Betsy Houchen, JD, MS, RN, Executive Director, Ohio Board of Nursing; Richard Young, MBA, RN; Marion Wilson, RN; and Terry Tran, JD, RN.

The Panel acknowledges Ms. Kate Jones, Ms. Kelly Michale, and Mr. David Henley, Practice and Regulation Administrative Assistants, and extends special thanks to Barbara Blakney, MN, RN, President, American Nurses Association; and Marilyn Chow, PhD, RN, FAAN, The Joint Commission Board Member, for their thoughtful review of early versions of TERCAP® and for their wisdom in identifying the support needed from nursing organizations regarding this project.

Kathy Malloch
Chairperson
NCSBN Expert Panel on Practice Breakdown

Overview: NCSBN Practice Breakdown Initiative

Kathy Malloch ◆ *Patricia Benner* ◆ *Vickie Sheets* ◆ *Kevin Kenward* ◆
Marie Farrell

Chapter Outline

*Everyone can recall lessons learned from experience. Often the best remembered lessons are the ones that were hardest learned—gleaned from making mistakes and dealing with the fallout from those mistakes. By studying situations where nursing practice breaks down, nurses can learn from the experiences of their colleagues. This is far better than learning from reliving the same difficult experiences (**Author Unknown**).*

Each day, in most health care settings in the United States, nurses monitor and manage the health care patients receive. The goal of these efforts is to ensure that the health care team delivers high-quality and safe patient care. Despite these efforts, missteps occur as do undetected changes in patients' conditions. These missteps and undetected changes are cause for great concern, and they challenge caregivers to examine their practices, and to create safer practices and ultimately better patient outcomes. The traditional, punitive, blame-placing practices that are found in most health care organizations also give cause for great concern, as those involved in these missteps are often reluctant to report them.

For these reasons (and others described below), the National Council of State Boards of Nursing (NCSBN) launched a national initiative in 1999 entitled the Practice Breakdown Advisory Panel (PBAP). The objective of the PBAP was to study nursing practice breakdown, to identify common themes related to those events, and most importantly, to recommend strategies to individuals, teams, and organizations to correct unsafe conditions and practices. This work would then assist boards of nursing to shift the focus from blame and punishment to prevention, remediation, and correction. Punishment would be limited to those cases of willful negligence and misconduct.

Since its inception, the PBAB has worked with representatives from its 60 member boards and with its consultant, Dr. Patricia Benner, to develop an initial minimum data set on practice breakdown reported to state boards of nursing. The goal was to develop an instrument that can distinguish human and system errors from willful negligence and intentional misconduct, while identifying the area of actual nursing practice breakdown in relation to core goals and standards of good nursing practice. An additional and equally important aim was to serve as a guide to increase the skills and competence of regulatory professionals in addressing practice breakdowns.

GOALS OF THE INITIATIVE

The goals of studying practice breakdown are to develop a consistent approach to assessing patient safety and reporting errors that will increase knowledge and incentives for error detection, reporting, and prevention while fulfilling the duty to protect the public from unsafe practices. These goals constitute a paradigm shift that reframes the focus from the individual, the nurse, to one that emphasizes prevention and the implications for the health care system, the health care team, and the individual nurse. The mechanism for achieving these goals was to create a standardized data collection instrument for investigators throughout the United States who carry responsibility for examining incidents of practice breakdown. The instrument, described below, is entitled Taxonomy of Error, Root Cause Analysis, and Practice Responsibility, or "TERCAP®." The PBAP also created additional products and initiatives that are discussed in this chapter.

FOCUS OF THE BOOK

This book presents an overview of the work that the NCSBN has undertaken to assist others committed to improving patient safety. The elements of this initiative include a framework for analyzing practice breakdown, the data collection instrument TERCAP, and selected tools and practices to implement its use.

This framework and ways of thinking about practice breakdown are useful not only for boards of nursing but also for nursing students, faculty, nurses in practice, hospital and other health care administrators, and other accrediting and regulatory agencies that oversee and support the practice of nursing. It is expected that this framework and way of thinking will also be useful to policy makers and those developing, refining, and reframing nurse practice acts. Finally, this work provides the evidence and creates an infrastructure for a major change in the way nurses conceptualize and manage practice breakdown.

PATIENT SAFETY: A DEFINITION

Cooper et al. (2000) describe patient safety as "... the avoidance, prevention, and improvement of adverse outcomes or injuries stemming from the processes of health care (errors, deviations, accidents) ..." (National Patient Safety Foundation, 1999, pp. 1-2) and suggest that improving safety depends on learning the ways in which safety emerges from interactions of the components. Woods calls for "... research that matters ... to identify critical success factors by moving beyond morbidity and mortality (dedicating a) larger role to functional status, caregiver burden, satisfaction with care, costs of care and cost-effectiveness" (Woods, 2004).

RATIONALE FOR THE INITIATIVE

Members of the NCSBN have expressed, for quite some time, concerns about the lack of evidence for the discipline and began to examine discipline practices from an anecdotal perspective in the 1990s. Concern persisted for the value of board sanctions such as probationary mandates, official censure, and nondisciplinary letters and their relationship to nurse behavior. Board members and staff are uncertain about whether the discipline imposed provided the intervention to effect improvement in practice behavior. The PBAP was formed in 1999 because of these concerns. Further, around this time, the Institute of Medicine (IOM) began publishing its work on patient safety.

INSTITUTE OF MEDICINE REPORT

There have always been medical and nursing errors, and these errors have always been of concern to both practitioners and patients. In 1998 the IOM captured the attention of both the media and the public when it published its landmark report *To Err Is Human* (Kohn et al., 2000) and identified the pervasive reality of errors related to health care. Since then, patient safety has become an overriding concern of the public at large, and some characterize this concern as a crisis of faith.

The IOM produced a second report in the fall of 2004 entitled *Keeping Patients Safe: Transforming the Work Environment of Nurses* (Page, 2004). Several aspects of the report include implications for research in practice breakdown. Of particular interest is Recommendation 7-2.

> The NCSBN, in consultation with patient safety experts and health care leaders, should undertake an initiative to design uniform processes across states to better distinguish human errors from willful negligence and intentional misconduct, along with guidelines for their application by state boards of nursing and other state regulatory bodies having authority over nursing (Page, 2004).

In the United States, the most appropriate place to examine this phenomenon would occur at the state level, through the state boards of nursing. This is because these boards are charged with the task of addressing key issues that are informed by the principles that guide their actions.

THE WORK OF BOARDS OF NURSING

The work of boards of nursing in the United States is complex for several reasons:

1. The primary obligation of boards of nursing is to protect the public through effective delineation of the scope of practice, licensure, certification, and discipline.
2. The public/patient should be protected from unsafe institutional design and policies that impede or prohibit safe, effective nursing care. Boards of nursing must distinguish between system, individual, and practice issues before determining the actual violation of a nurse practice act. For example, organizational system processes within health care settings often result in suboptimal or even forced choices between competing justified needs and demands of good patient care. Negative outcomes for some patients may come at the expense of meeting the crisis or emergency intervention requirements of other patients.
3. Evidence for effective professional accountability needs to be established. Effective decision-making results when the nurse recognizes the fiduciary/advocacy responsibility she/he has for the patient and is able to meet those responsibilities by adequate safe institutional design, orientation, and ongoing in-service education, staffing, and policies.

CUTBACKS, NURSING SHORTAGES, REDUCED HOSPITAL STAYS

Suboptimal institutional environments impede safe patient care. Many complex elements have contributed to this current crisis of faith in the health care system. Specifically, these elements in the form of errors came to the forefront as health care institutions implemented cutbacks in nurse-patient staffing ratios, increased nursing workload, overtime, and temporary employees. These cutbacks were exacerbated by the trend of shorter hospital stays for patients who were acutely ill and, in turn, some of the checks and balances that helped ensure patient safety were also eliminated. The nursing shortage further complicates the situation. This is partly because the complexity that results from reduced time for hospital stays and its concomitant compressed time allotment requires not only more nurses but nurses with higher levels of competence to assess, synthesize, and coordinate patient care needs.

CREATING A FAIR AND JUST HEALTH CARE CULTURE

Concerned health care organizations have recognized the complexity of these trends and their impact on practice breakdown. They worked to shift a health care culture that emphasized blaming the individual to one that looked to improve performance of the system and to reduce systems errors. Some experts have called for a no-blame culture as the solution to the problems resulting from fear and intimidation from error management. Much has been written about these no-blame cultures, viewed as a key mechanism to reduce errors and as an approach to what has evolved as a patient safety movement.

Most health care professionals recognize that shame, blame, and punishment for mistakes do not improve patient safety. In many situations, patient safety is compromised as situations are not fully analyzed and corrected for fear of further punishment. Many now recognize that a nonconstructive position is one in which an either-or position is taken—that is, where either the individual or the system is determined to be at fault, or where the system is always at fault and the individual is the victim. Rather, the desired expectation is a culture characterized by fairness and justice.

A *just culture* for practice breakdown management is one in which the reality of the environment, organizational cultures, and missteps are viewed as critical learning opportunities for patient safety, while also addressing carelessness, inattentiveness, and substandard practice as well as intentional misconduct in any work environment (Marx, 2001). The goal is to avoid the tendency to blame individuals for patient safety issues when the error is unintentional and is usually a product of many forces and mishaps that led to the practice breakdown. However, a just culture demands attention, repair, remediation, and discipline of those professionals who willfully ignore their professional standards. A just culture requires mutual support for a difficult and complex job, accountability for meeting the standards of good practice by all workers, and rigorous attempts to protect the public from unsafe practices. An additional goal is to avoid the tendency to blame individuals for patient safety issues when, in fact, more factors are involved than one person's actions alone. Shared practice responsibility is a critical consideration in addition to separate considerations of the individual and the health care system's contributions to practice breakdown.

An oppositional argument about *either an individual or a systems approach* is wrongheaded, since both are required in addition to carrying out the notions of good and upholding the standards of good practice of any person who is a licensed professional (Benner et al., 2002; Page, 2004). Such an oppositional view usually posits the individual as an isolated individual rather than a member-participant of a professional practice community that has publicly made a commitment to uphold the notions of good and standards of a particular profession. If the individual imagined is a competitive individual (as in an extremely competitive business model), then there can be no accounting for the moral sources and collective standards of practice, commitment to good practice, skilled know-how, ethos, and participation in the formative outcomes of an accredited professional educational program. Accrediting bodies such as the State Board of Registered Nurses accredit schools of nursing for imparting skilled know-how, knowledge of the discipline, and ethical comportment, which includes both self-improving practice and safe practice. Rather than thinking of the individual as self-maximizing or competitive, in a professional practice one needs to think of professionals (nurses, doctors, lawyers, clergy, etc.) as *members-participants* of the profession, committed to the notions of good internal to the practice (MacIntyre, 1984) and formed by their educational processes to have a fiduciary responsibility to their patients, clients, and parishioners.

Yet, Page (2004) and her colleagues point out:

> ...An extreme systems perspective that recognizes no individual contributions to patient safety presents problems such as "learned helplessness" and failure to address instances of individual deficits in competencies or willful wrongdoing.

> With regard to the phenomenon "learned helplessness" . . .health care practitioners may be tempted to lessen their personal vigilance and striving for personal excellence and think, "It's the system—there is nothing I can do about it." But safe and effective care depends upon each professional continuing the struggle under less-than-ideal local circumstances (Reason, 1997 [as cited by Page, 2004, p. 31]).

If it were possible to make medicine absolutely scientific technical certainties with no unresearched aspects and no great individual variations in patients or in diseases/injuries, then a closed system designed to be "error free" would be possible, as is the case for manufacturing processes that are functioning well under tightly controlled circumstances. But medicine and nursing require professionals who are well educated, skillful, and ethically committed to patients' well-being because professional skill and judgment are required, even as the best scientific evidence for practice is used. Medical and nursing clinical situations, unlike well-controlled manufacturing processes, are underdetermined, open ended, and highly variable, and therefore require highly professional judgment and skilled know-how by nurses and physicians who are committed to act well on behalf of the patient's best interests. Systems in health care delivery are open systems. In health care, systems engineering focuses on the structures, processes, and functions of an open living system in relation to inputs and outcomes. Constant input related to knowledge, science, skill, repair, and redesign is needed for open systems. Systems analysis captures what has already happened as a result of system failure or breakdown; therefore systems repair is post hoc related to a past failure, and future oriented in designing a better system to prevent future similar failures. Professional practice communities are required to shore up and prevent immediate failure or intervene immediately in a present practice breakdown. All human systems require ongoing repair and redesign by individuals and practice communities who work together to sustain a self-improving practice.

As technology proliferates and makes work less transparent, so does the likelihood for new types of errors (Page, 2004; Reason, 1990). It is no longer possible for any one clinician to know and/or remember all the needed information for practice as noted by the *Quality Chasm Report* (Committee on the Quality of Health Care in America, 2001):

> Today, no one clinician can retain all the information necessary for sound, evidence-based practice. No unaided human being can read, recall, and act effectively on the volume of clinically relevant scientific literature (pp. 44-45). Relying on memory has become a hazard for patient safety as the amount and complexity of information continues to grow. Nurses need to be aided with information systems and decision aid systems (Page, 2004).

SHARED PRACTICE RESPONSIBILITY

All professions have the responsibility to be self-regulating and self-improving. All member participants of a professional practice have a shared public and civic responsibility to uphold the standards of the practice and to practice in such a way as to ensure ongoing improvement in the practice. Professional practice is never upheld by one individual practitioner alone. It relies in part on institutional conditions to enable good practice through system level infrastructures and organizational planning and integrity. It also relies on cooperation and collaborative effort among health care professionals who live up to the notions and standards of good practice. Complex professional practice relies on ethical, knowledge-based, and skillful practice by professionals who use clinical judgment in underdetermined clinical situations. Practice communities develop and share local practice knowledge, standards, and norms, and uphold these as members of both the local professional practice community and their larger professional communities of nursing or medicine.

The professional practice of nursing is a socially organized discipline in which its participants have been educated and tested for licensure. Professional nurses carry responsibilities to each other and to other health care team members to uphold the notions of good practice. They hold these standards of good practice in common within nursing and with other interdisciplinary team members such as physicians, pharmacists, respiratory therapists, and social workers. Professionals, by definition, have entered into a covenant to act as responsible, professional citizen members in education, licensure, and practice and through participation in professional associations (Sullivan, 2004; 2005).

The PBAP considers these professional dimensions and the relationships among the individual, the health care team, and the health care system. These elements interact in ways that honor and integrate self-governing, socially organized practice members who work professionally to participate in the everyday practices of a health care delivery team. However, a serious oversight occurs when these relationships and shared professional talents and commitments are not considered in an examination of errors. Reporting and preventing errors in any profession are serious expectations for all members of self-improving professional practice. Professional practice is impossible without these shared expectations.

THE DESIRED OUTCOME

Administrators and leaders need to support health care cultures that value questioning practices, collaborating on challenges to the health care team, and pursuing activities to promote professional development. Woods described the "holy grail [of research] that everyone wants but no one has" to include:

1. A measure of nurses' work
2. Descriptive studies of nursing-related error
3. Safer and more effective work processes and work spaces (supported by information technology)
4. A standardized approach to measuring patient acuity
5. Safe staffing levels based on outcomes in different types of nursing units
6. Effects of successive workdays/sustained work hours on patient safety
7. Descriptive studies of levels of education, preparation, and outcomes
8. Models of collaborative care, including care by multidisciplinary teams (Woods, 2004)

BOARDS OF NURSING AS SOURCES OF DATA

Boards of nursing possess a potentially rich source of data that could examine sources of nursing error and thus are well positioned to add to the body of knowledge surrounding this aspect of health care errors. This is, in part, because the kinds of errors typically reported to boards of nursing are usually serious in nature, and the knowledge from these examinations provides descriptive studies of nursing-related error. Further, the data from these studies hold great potential for developing more effective strategies to prevent and reduce serious errors at the institutional and professional practice levels.

Boards of nursing have access to data from educational and service settings. Board members can examine aggregate data and the disciplinary actions that arise from both of these settings. These reviews provide a more complex but meaningful set of data than if the service setting or the educational setting alone were the focus of examination. By studying practice breakdown, boards can promote patient safety and prevention of error by identifying nurses and nursing situations *at risk* for potential practice breakdowns. This new preventive regulatory role promotes proactive regulation before harm occurs rather than waiting to discipline after problems are reported.

Under the supervision and quality control of the NCSBN, this national database of nursing errors reported to state boards of nursing could become a source of additional research studies conducted by researchers, including graduate students, who want to examine practice breakdown and patient safety. For example, an outside researcher might want to focus on errors associated with the administration of medications or practice breakdown episodes related to nursing interventions, either failure to intervene or inappropriate intervention. Any of the elements or all areas of nursing practice areas could be compared locally, regionally, and nationally in order to better understand the causes of practice breakdown in nursing. This database could also shed light on a particular state's or a particular type of institution's comparisons of errors and patient harm with the national database. The NCSBN will encourage such outside research projects, and provide oversight and quality control as such studies evolve.

By going public and making the regulatory work of state boards of nursing more transparent to staff nurses and student nurses, the NCSBN hopes to encourage primary prevention of practice breakdown and draw attention to the central role of safety work that has long been a hallmark of nursing practice (Benner, Hooper-Kyriakidis, & Stannard, 1999). By systematically understanding the regulatory functions of the nursing profession and the major kinds of errors that nurses are likely to be involved in at some point in their careers, nurses will be better prepared to respond appropriately to practice breakdown through accurate documentation, reporting, truth telling, and immediate measures to minimize harm to the patient. The situations reported to the state boards of nursing are typically more harmful to patients, fall outside the standards of good practice, involve knowledge-skill deficits, and in those ways differ significantly from errors that would never be reported to state boards of nursing. For example, the following medication error that occurred early in the nursing career of Dianne Pestolesi, who was on the nursing faculty (Benner et al., in press), is a classic kind of error that would not be reported to the state board because the nurse took all the appropriate actions, notified the physician immediately, addressed the potential harm to the patient by altering her care, and successfully prevented the potential harm to her patient:

> I was to give Synthroid IV to a woman who was hypothyroid. I thought the order was a very large dose. When the vials came up there were three vials to be reconstituted, which again made me think that this is too large of a dose, so I called the pharmacy and the pharmacist said, "Well it is a large dose, but it is within the possible range of dosages." I had this icky feeling that it wasn't right. I went to the patient and as I was pushing the IV med in, again, I had this icky feeling that it was the wrong dose. So I then went back to the chart and looked at the doctor's order, which I had not done, but should have done from the beginning. And it was an error. I had given the patient three times the amount of the drug that was intended. I went hot and cold. I thought well this is the end of my nursing career! I would lose my license. I called the doctor and told him about the error. "I am really sorry; I have made a terrible medication error. I gave your patient three times the dosage of Synthroid that was ordered. What can I do to help this patient? He said to watch her closely for arrhythmias and to carry Inderal in my pocket, ready to administer it to her if she had a tachycardia. I arranged with the other nurses to watch my other patients while I stayed in the patient's room. The patient became very antsy, and very hot then, for the first time after surgery needed to have a bowel movement. The patient dramatized all the symptoms of hyperthyroid. I fanned the patient. I put a cool cloth on her head, and stayed with her. Her pulse stayed below 120. She came through it without arrhythmias, but I will never give the wrong dose of Synthroid again. I will always check the original order and call the doctor if I have questions. I will never go against my instincts, overriding my icky feeling that this is not right. I learned that I could survive and continue to be a nurse, even though I made a terrible error. I am grateful that the patient came through OK. I filled out an incident report at the end of the shift (Benner et al., Chapter 4, in press).

Ms. Dianne Pestolesi, RN, MSN, now tells this story to her students as a cautionary tale. She is equally vivid in describing her own foreboding and fears for the patient, and the patient's actual responses. She acted responsibly and took responsibility for *learning* from her error. She points out to her students that she now attends to the usual match between range of dose and packaging of the medication. She was a newly graduated nurse when this incident occurred and did not yet attend to her growing practical experiential knowledge. She models for her students the most ethical response to an error. She made no effort to hide her mistake, which always compounds any error and increases the consequences for making the error. If the patient, public, and health care team members cannot trust the accuracy of documentation of care given and doses of medication given, then the patient is placed in a situation of potential further harm. Wu (2000) proclaims that providers who make an error, particularly an error that causes harm, are "the second victim" of the error.

In the context of a "shame and blame" culture, errors are more likely to be covered over, and the one committing the error is tempted to remain silent and avoid telling the patient (Wu et al., 1991). However, all these responses lack integrity and expose the patient and health care team—including the one making the error—to even more harm. Had Dianne Pestolesi covered up her error, not called the physician, and not charted this overdose, she likely would have been reported to the state board of nursing for endangering a patient. She herself would have become a victim of guilt and remorse. While she regretted her error, she took steps to avoid ever making the same mistake again by honestly reporting the error immediately and following through with protective attentive care of her patient until she was through the resulting "thyroid storm" of the high dosage. She now uses her example to let students know that everyone can and will make an error without intending to, and responding with integrity is the only possible way forward.

It is impossible to prevent all errors. Members of highly reliable organizations who also engage in high-risk work imagine all the possible pitfalls and errors that might occur (Weick & Sutcliffe, 2001). This turns out to increase the reliability of performance when it spurs persons in the highly reliable organization to imagine and correct potential errors and to take seriously and act preventively when "near misses" occur. It is an opposite response to a culture of low expectations (Reason, 1990; Wachter, 2008; Wachter & Shojania, 2004) where mistakes such as misspelling of patient names, misidentification, or underreporting of procedures are common and thus commonly overlooked as a basis for further checking. This book will contain many actual cases and cautionary tales that we hope will assist staff nurses, administrators, and student nurses in preventing recurrence of the kinds of practice breakdowns that commonly occur in nursing.

This book seeks to augment the excellent educational initiative to improve the education of undergraduate and graduate nurses about improving patient safety, sponsored by the Robert Wood Johnson Foundation and led by Linda Cronenwett. This project, Quality and Safety Education for Nurses (QSEN) (www.QSEN.org), seeks to improve education in quality improvement and patient safety in nursing education. Cronenwett and colleagues (Cronenwett et al., 2007) acknowledge that patient safety is firmly lodged in the nursing tradition and summarize some of the goals of their project as follows:

> At the core of nursing lies incredible historical will to ensure quality and safety for patients. Many current endeavors, such as the work occurring in the Robert Wood Johnson Foundation–sponsored project, *Transforming Care at the Bedside*, demonstrate how quality/safety/improvement work attracts the hearts of nurses, resulting in the "joy in work"[1] Developing health professionals capable of continually improving health care quality, safety and value: The health professional educator's work[1] that retains the health care workforce. Attending to the development of QSEN competencies may help nurses—who love the basic work of nursing—love their *jobs,* too (Cronenwett et al., 2007, p. 122).

---

[1]Batalden, P. (2005). Developing health professionals capable of continually improving health care quality, safety and value: The health professional educator's work. Available at http://www.QSEN.org. Accessed October 22, 2008.

TABLE **1.1** Institute Of Medicine Competencies

PATIENT-CENTERED CARE

Definition: Recognize the patient or designee as the source of control and full partner in providing compassionate and coordinated care based on respect for patient's preferences, values, and needs
http://qsen.org/competencydomains/teamwork-and-collaboration/

TEAMWORK AND COLLABORATION

Definition: Function effectively within nursing and interprofessional teams, fostering open communication, mutual respect, and shared decision-making to achieve quality patient care

EVIDENCE-BASED PRACTICE

Definition: Integrate best current evidence with clinical expertise and patient/family preferences and values for delivery of optimal health care

QUALITY IMPROVEMENT

Definition: Use data to monitor the outcomes of care processes and use improvement methods to design and test changes to continuously improve the quality and safety of health care systems

SAFETY

Definition: Minimizes risk of harm to patients and providers through both system effectiveness and individual performance

INFORMATICS

Definition: Use information and technology to communicate, manage knowledge, mitigate error, and support decision making

Table 1.1 lists the definitions of the IOM competencies for nursing and the knowledge skills and attitudes that were developed in the QSEN project for curricula in undergraduate nursing based on these competencies.

CONCEPTUAL FRAMEWORK

In developing the nursing taxonomy of error, we inductively identified nursing practice breakdowns that were reported to a state board of nursing that were considered to fall within the very general rubric of "clinical judgment." Because this rubric proved to be so inclusive in an earlier classification study conducted by the state board, and because there was particular diversity and challenge in developing the range of corrective measures that were required for this very large category of nursing practice breakdown, we decided to inductively generate a taxonomy of nursing practice breakdown within reported cases that had been classified as breakdowns in clinical judgment in the past. Working back and forth from commonly held notions of good nursing practice and the cases of practice breakdown, the PBAB generated the categories of nursing practice breakdown based on breakdowns in usual standards of good nursing practice, which inherently contain areas of patient safety work The·conceptual framework that informed this study focuses on the aspects of nursing practice to which nurses attend when care is planned, practiced, and evaluated as expected (Table 1.2). Within these three, the following standards of good nursing practice are identified.

SAFE MEDICATION ADMINISTRATION

The nurse administers the right dose of the right medication via the right route to the right patient at the right time for the right reason.

DOCUMENTATION

Nursing documentation provides relevant information about the patient and the measures implemented in response to their needs.

ATTENTIVENESS/SURVEILLANCE

The nurse monitors what is happening with the patient and staff. The nurse observes the patient's clinical condition; if the nurse has not observed a patient, then he/she cannot identify changes if they occurred and/or make knowledge-able discernments and decisions about the patient.

TABLE **1.2 Patient-Centered Care**

Definition: Recognize patient or designee as source of control and full partner in providing compassionate and coordinated care based on respect for patient's preferences, values, and needs

Knowledge	Skills	Attitudes
Integrate understanding of multiple dimensions of patient centered care: • Patient/family/community preferences, values • Coordination and integration of care • Information, communication, and education • Physical comfort and emotional support • Involvement of family and friends • Transition and continuity	Elicit patient values, preferences, and expressed needs as part of clinical interview, implementation of care plan, and evaluation of care Communicate patient values, preferences, and expressed needs to other members of health care team	Value seeing health care situations "through patients' eyes" Respect and encourage individual expression of patient values, preferences, and expressed needs Value the patient's expertise with own health and symptoms

Continued

TABLE **1.2** Patient-Centered Care—Cont'd

Knowledge	Skills	Attitudes
Describe how diverse cultural, ethnic, and social backgrounds function as sources of patient, family, and community values	Provide patient-centered care with sensitivity and respect for the diversity of human experience	Seek learning opportunities with patients who represent all aspects of human diversity Recognize personally held attitudes about working with patients from different ethnic, cultural, and social backgrounds Willingly support patient-centered care for individuals and groups whose values differ from own
Demonstrate comprehensive understanding of concepts of pain and suffering, including physiologic models of pain and comfort.	Assess presence and extent of pain and suffering Assess levels of physical and emotional comfort	Recognize personally held values and beliefs about management of pain or suffering
	Elicit expectations of patient and family for relief of pain, discomfort, or suffering	Appreciate role of the nurse in relief of all types and sources of pain or suffering
	Initiate effective treatments to relieve pain and suffering in light of patient values, preferences, and expressed needs	Recognize that patient expectations influence outcomes in management of pain or suffering

CLINICAL REASONING

Nurses interpret patients' signs, symptoms, and responses to therapies. Nurses evaluate the relevance of changes in patient signs and symptoms, and ensure that patient care providers are notified and patient care is adjusted appropriately. All nursing care requires clinical judgment, but for the purposes of capturing errors related to clinical judgment, this work limits the definition of practice breakdown associated with clinical reasoning to those events related to inadequate titration and adjustment of therapies and therapeutic actions based on the patient's responses to those therapies. The attempt is to capture the increasing importance of nurses' adjustment and titration of therapies based on the patient's responses.

PREVENTION

The nurse follows usual and customary measures to prevent risks, hazards, or complications due to illness or hospitalization. These include fall precautions, preventing hazards of immobility, contractures, stasis pneumonia, and more.

INTERVENTION

The nurse properly carries out nursing actions.

INTERPRETATION OF AUTHORIZED PROVIDER ORDERS

The nurse interprets and translates into action authorized provider orders.

PROFESSIONAL RESPONSIBILITY/PATIENT ADVOCACY

The nurse demonstrates professional responsibility and understands the nature of the nurse-patient relationship. Advocacy refers to the expectations that a nurse acts responsibly in protecting patient/family vulnerabilities and in advocating to see that patient needs or concerns are addressed (Benner et al., 2006).

It is both notable and understandable that these inductively generated areas of nursing practice are all central to both the occurrence and prevention of patient care breakdown since nursing practice has a long tradition of patient safety work as central to the everyday nursing practice (Benner, Hooper-Kyriakidis, & Stannard, 1999).

Prior to the development of the report *Keeping Patients Safe: Transforming the Work Environment of Nurses* (Page, 2004), the focus had been on epidemiology of health care errors and quality improvement in the safety for systems of delivery of health care (Aspden et al., 2004, 2006; Committee on the Quality of Health Care in America, 2001; Greiner & Knebel, 2001; Kohn, Corrigan, & Donaldson, 2000). In 2004 (Page, 2004), the focus was on the problematic work environments of nurses, environments that often force errors through short staffing, excessive work overtime, frequent interruptions of nurses' work, lack of use of informatics focused on safety, high pressure for efficiency and productivity, and so on. Stone et al. (2007) examined the relationship between nurse staffing and hospital characteristics and specific patient safety measures, such as nosocomial infection rates and incidence of decubitus ulcers. They found that higher nurse-to-patient ratios and increased overtime diminished patient safety outcomes and increased in-hospital mortality rates. TERCAP seeks to capture aspects of the work environment that contribute to nursing practice breakdown.

The safety work of nurses and physicians is intertwined, and their roles often overlap. But the focus and clinical "know-how" of the two professions remain as a built-in cross-check for patients when the work and health care team cultures are collaborative and synergistic. For example, the success of "checklist" strategies for improving patient safety often rely on physician and nursing performance, but the nurse who typically has more continuous time with the patient and in the health care delivery setting is the key to making checklists work on a daily basis. Gawande, in an article published in *The New Yorker* in 2007, points to Peter Pronovost's efforts and demonstrated success in improving quality of patient care through the use of checklists. Checklists deal with forgetfulness and the hazards of relying on memory for everyday performance of routine safety and quality work. Often health care providers do not understand the safety and quality implications inherent to protocols, and thus skip them. Gawande (2007) describes nurses' contributions to the success of the use of patient safety checklists:

> One [Checklist] aimed to insure that nurses observe patients for pain at least once every four hours and provide timely pain medication. This reduced the likelihood of a patient's experiencing untreated pain from 41% to 3%. [Another tested checklist ensured] the head of each patient's bed was propped up at least thirty degrees so that oral secretions couldn't go into the windpipe, and antacid medication was given to prevent stomach ulcers.[2] The proportion of patients who didn't receive the recommended care dropped from 70% to 4%; the occurrence of pneumonias fell by a quarter; and 21 fewer patients died than in the previous year. The researchers found that simply having the doctors and nurses in the I.C.U. make their own checklists for what they thought should be done each day improved the consistency of care to the point that, within a few weeks, the average length of patient stay in intensive care dropped by half (p. 5).

Gawande also points out that it was the nurses who monitored the checklists, keeping them current and effective.

Gawande's (2007) article points out the increasingly central role that nurses play in quality improvement and patient safety. He also points to the challenges of increasing complexity in nursing, and medicine has compounded the problems with safety work in the hospital. Nurses in acute care settings, and particularly in intensive care units, have many exposures to risks of errors daily because of the number of patient interventions they perform daily.

---

[2]Since the writing of this chapter, antacids in the form of proton-pump inhibitors have been found to increase ventilator acquired pneumonia by 30%. Herzig, S.J., Howell, M.D., Marcantonio, E.R. (2009). Acid-suppressive medication use and the risk for hospital-acquired pneumonia. *JAMA 301*(20): 2120-8.

Practice breakdown is the disruption or absence of any of the aspects of good practice. It occurs when individuals, the health care team, or the health care system do not attend to one or more of these central aspects of nursing practice that each contribute to patient safety and quality improvement work.

Reason (1990) provided a way to think about errors at the organizational and systems levels. When weak points and holes within an organizational system line up, errors occur more often. For example, a hierarchical system with steep lines of authority and emphasis on top-down one-way communication creates a system that is prone to errors. Add production pressures, lack of procedures to double-check patient identification, or read back plans for verification, along with a "culture of low expectation" ("people often get it wrong here, nothing unusual to worry about, no further checking is warranted") can line up much like holes in a stack of Swiss cheese. The error did not start out to be an error, but it was supported by a careless aggregation of lack of safety checks, poor communication, and time pressure.

Reason's model was derived from many accident studies in aviation, nuclear power, and complex organizations. He pointed to the importance of seeing the multiple layers of Swiss cheese with large holes, the large holes indicating lack of multiple layers of protection and poor safety system design. A focus on the individual alone at the sharp end of the error parallels the days before automobiles were designed for safety. The driver was admonished to drive carefully in a dangerously designed device that had no built-in protection systems such as air bags, safety belts, roll bars, and so forth. The holes in the system can be considered the root cause of the conditions for the possibility of the error.

We followed Charles Vincent's framework for root cause analysis in identifying the system contributions to errors. Vincent's framework is displayed in Table 1.3. We included Vincent's institutional organization and management;

TABLE 1.3 Framework of Factors Influencing Clinical Practice and Contributing to Adverse Effects*

Framework	Contributory Factors	Examples of Problems That Contribute to Errors
Institutional	Regulatory content Medicolegal environment	Insufficient priority given by regulators to safety issues; legal pressures against open discussion, preventing the opportunity to learn from adverse events
Organization and management	Financial resources and constraints Policy standards and goals Safety culture and priorities	Lack of awareness of safety issues on the part of senior management; policies leading to inadequate staffing levels

Continued

TABLE 1.3 Framework of Factors Influencing Clinical Practice and Contributing to Adverse Effects*—Cont'd

Framework	Contributory Factors	Examples of Problems That Contribute to Errors
Work environment	Staffing levels and mix of skills Patterns in workload and shift Design, availability, and maintenance of equipment Administrative and managerial support	Heavy workloads, leading to fatigue; limited access to essential equipment; inadequate administrative support, leading to reduced time with patients
Team	Verbal communication Written communication Supervision and willingness to seek help Team leadership	Poor supervision of junior staff; poor communication among different professions; unwillingness of junior staff to seek assistance
Individual staff member	Knowledge and skills Motivation and attitude Physical and mental health	Lack of knowledge or experience; long-term fatigue and stress
Task	Availability and use of protocols Availability and accuracy of test results	Unavailability of test results or delay in obtaining them; lack of clear protocols and guidelines
Patient	Complexity and seriousness of condition Language and communication Personality and social factors	Distress; language barriers between patients and caregivers

*Based on Vincent et al. (1998). Framework for analyzing risk and safety in clinical medicine. *BMJ, 316*(7138), 1154-1157.

work environment, team, individual staff member(s) task, and patient in the TERCAP instrument (see *TERCAP*, available at www.NCSBN.org).

We anticipate that as patient safety and quality improvement develops, revisions and additions to TERCAP will be made. Eventually we will need to consider the evidence on the best practices for patient safety and quality improvement. For example, I-SBAR (an acronym that stands for Introduction of caregivers and patients; Situation—a brief statement of the problem; Background relevant for the situation at hand, Assessment—summary of what the clinician believes is the underlying cause and its severity, and Recommendation—what is needed to resolve the situation) (Pope, Rodzen, & Spross, 2008) has been shown to be successful in reducing communication barriers when used by rapid response teams and is promoted by the Institute for Healthcare Improvement as a communication method (IHI website, http://www.ihi.org/ihi). Nurses are in an excellent position to evaluate the use of quality improvement measures designed to improve communication and strategies such as checklists to ensure continuity and consistency among the health care team in performing patient safety protocols.

STUDY QUESTIONS

The PBAP was created to facilitate the exploration in the future of the following study questions based on the definition of safety and the conceptual framework of the study:

1. What patient characteristics are associated with different types of practice breakdown?
2. What nurse characteristics (demographic data) are associated with different types of practice breakdown?
3. What scheduling, staffing levels, and timing of incidents are associated with different types of practice breakdown?
4. Which nurses of different licensure types are associated with different types of practice breakdown?
5. What educational characteristics are associated with different types of practice breakdown?
6. What types of health care institutions are associated with different types of practice breakdown?
7. What types of health care system factors are associated with different types of practice breakdown?
8. What types of health care team factors are associated with different types of practice breakdown?
9. What clusters of practice breakdown are associated with primary nursing types of error?
10. What types of practice breakdown are associated with patient harm?
11. What types of patient medical record documentation are associated with different types of practice breakdown?

OPERATIONAL DEFINITIONS

The PBAP developed and used a set of operational definitions (see *TERCAP Code Book,* available at www.NCSBN.org).

ASSUMPTIONS

The PBAP assumed that:
1. Data were collected by investigators that included nurses and non-nurses.
2. Confidentiality of all records would be maintained in accordance with national and state policies.
3. Data were collected and integrated within the context of the investigator's customary and usual intake processes.
4. Data were collected through electronic entry.
5. Data were reported accurately and honestly.
6. The data collection instrument developed would not *add* a document to the current process; rather, it would enhance and integrate the existing system of inquiry.

SETTING

The setting for this study was the health care practice settings within the jurisdictions of state boards of nursing throughout the United States. The PBAP collected data regarding the development of TERCAP during a pilot study conducted between April and May 2005.

STUDY DESIGN

The PBAP's goal was to create a valid, reliable, standardized, data collection instrument that investigators would use to examine practice breakdown and error in the health care workplace. The initial challenge was to identify the major types of nursing practice breakdown and to create a taxonomy of these distinct kinds of practice breakdown, and to examine causes common to situations in which safety was at risk and in which error occurred. Such a taxonomy overlaps with a "A Taxonomy of Medical Errors Made by Physicians," described in Table 1.4, but has additional types of error related particularly to nursing care.

The research design included a qualitative descriptive case study analysis over a period of 6 years and four reviews of actual cases at the state level. The PBAP derived the taxonomy through repeated analyses of 109 cases and identified 10 sections that informed the parts of the data collection instrument TERCAP (see *TERCAP,* available at www.NCSBN.org). The research design subsequently

TABLE **1.4** Taxonomy of Medical Errors for Physicians

TYPES OF ERRORS

Diagnostic
- Error or delay in diagnosis
- Failure to use indicated tests
- Use of outmoded tests or therapy
- Failure to act on results of monitoring or testing

Treatment
- Error in the performance of an operation, procedure, or test
- Error in administering the treatment
- Error in the dose or method of using a drug
- Avoidable delay in treatment or in responding to an abnormal test result
- Inappropriate (not indicated) care

Preventive
- Failure to provide prophylactic treatment
- Inadequate monitoring or follow-up treatment

Failure of communication

Equipment failure

Other system failures

Data from Leape, L.L., Lawthers, A.G., Brennan, T.A., Johnson, W.G. (1993). Preventing medical injury. *Quality Review Bulletin, 19*(5), 144-149.

included initial and follow-up assessments of TERCAP that resulted in documentation on the data collection instrument (described below).

SAMPLE

The membership of the PBAP was developed deliberately to include representatives of boards of nursing throughout the United States and an internationally recognized expert in the topic under investigation. Its membership was also designed to include nurses with expertise at the state level with extensive experience in dealing with practice breakdown. This expert panel reviewed the cases and used repeated examinations to establish the instrument's validity, reliability, and other essential qualities.

DATA COLLECTION INSTRUMENTS

PURPOSE AND DESCRIPTION

TERCAP is a 60-item electronic data collection instrument. Its purpose is to assist boards of nursing in collecting data using uniform processes across states to examine different patterns of errors and to distinguish practice breakdown from misconduct and willful negligence.

TERCAP: CASE STUDY ANALYSES

Initially, the PBAP analyzed 26 cases related to issues of discipline obtained from various jurisdictions to discover characteristics of nurses at risk for making errors and to learn more about practice breakdown. Ultimately, the expert panel examined 109 cases.

In the initial analyses, the PBAP examined documents that included original discipline complaints, investigative reports, additional relevant documentation, and public documents related to a case. When available, the analysis included the nurse's story in his or her own handwriting and/or transcripts of the nurse's interactions with the regulatory agency. Nurse and patient names were redacted from all materials prior to submission for analysis.

DESCRIPTION OF TERCAP

TERCAP is divided into 10 sections. The first section asks for information about the setting in which the practice breakdown occurred. This is to facilitate identification of multiple sources for error prevention. It also asks about the nurse's education, licensure, and work history.

Next, users are directed to identify in the next section the contributing elements of error. Investigators are invited to analyze the events of the case and determine the causes for practice breakdown. They select the primary cause of the breakdown from the taxonomy categories based on the category of breakdown they perceive as most proximal to causing the patient direct harm.

Data are also collected on other factors that may contribute to a discipline case. These include relevant practice and systems contributions to practice breakdown, outcomes for the involved patients, and outcomes related to the individual nurse. Finally, the investigators evaluate the outcomes of the case from the perspective of the patient and from the nurse.

VALIDITY

The PBAP used the data from the initial analysis to create and strengthen TERCAP for validity and reliability. They served as content experts as they examined early versions of TERCAP to track case elements and recurring themes, analysis of root cause, practitioner and health care team contributions, and practice responsibility. Subsequently they reviewed additional cases prior to finalizing the data collection instrument. Following these analyses, 16 boards of nursing submitted 109 cases using TERCAP. The PBAP's analysis identified problem areas and revised the data collection instrument based on these findings. In addition to these reviews, the president of the American Nurses Association (ANA) and a member of The Joint Commission reviewed the text and emphasized the need for a preventive rather than punitive focus.

The challenges of creating conceptual clarity for the eight categories of practice breakdown continually challenged the PBAP members. Definitions and clear descriptions of safe medication administration, documentation, prevention, and interventions emerged with little difficulty. The categories of attentiveness/surveillance, clinical reasoning, interpretation of provider orders, and professional advocacy/patient advocacy required much more discussion and clarification. Initially, the clinical reasoning category was labeled clinical judgment. This label proved to be too generic in that nursing practice requires clinical judgment in all patient care encounters. The term "clinical reasoning" was adopted to capture reasoning across time about changes in the patient's clinical condition and changes in the clinician's understanding of the patient's clinical condition (Benner, Hooper-Kyriakidis, & Stannard, 1999). Inherent to the narrower view of clinical reasoning is the adjustment of therapies administered by nurses according to the patient's responses so that a desirable therapeutic effect is achieved over time. Members further clarified the categories on a continuum basis. Attentiveness necessarily precedes clinical judgment. Once clinical judgment occurs, the next step is to intervene or provide care. Prevention follows clinical judgment since the nurse must determine the need for prevention prior to implementing preventive measures. Conceptual clarity about the aims and usual sequence of these eight practice breakdown categories improved inter-rater reliability among those using the TERCAP instrument.

The preparation of board investigators became an issue during the analysis of the cases. Although TERCAP was created from the perspective of nursing knowledge, many of the investigators at boards of nursing do not have nursing backgrounds. In light of this possible source of variance, the PBAP conducted additional revisions to ensure clarity for a broader group of investigators. Also the TERCAP code book was enriched with examples and operational definitions to guide the investigators' use of the TERCAP instrument.

RELIABILITY

Reliability is the extent to which different coders, each coding the same content, come to the same coding decisions. Data collection that relies on humans to obtain measurements involves estimates of agreement known as inter-rater reliability. Inter-rater reliability is used when opinions and interpretation of facts are required of multiple raters evaluating or interpreting the same behavior or information.

The need to establish inter-rater reliability is important for instruments such as TERCAP that are developed to evaluate the reasons practice breakdown occurs in the delivery of quality health care to patients. The TERCAP instrument requires the investigator to make a judgment about the patient's care and the nurse's behavior based on interviews and a review of records. The coder fills in the TERCAP instrument based on the facts of the case and on the investigator's interpretation of the event.

Many potential sources of measurement error may occur during this process. Inconsistency among raters regarding correct values or conclusions, bias, and idiosyncratic use of the instrument affects the reliability of the information provided. Establishing the degree of inter-rater reliability of a data collection instrument is a necessary condition before validity can be ascribed to the obtained set of ratings. If two or more coders cannot be shown to rate reliably, then any subsequent analyses of their ratings will yield false results.

To assess coder inter-rater reliability, several members of the expert panel created a hypothetical case study based on real cases and asked coders to complete TERCAP for the same case. Thirty-four people from boards of nursing, the NCSBN, and Practice Breakdown Advisory Panel (PBAP) read the case and completed TERCAP. Coders did not receive additional training on the latest version of the instrument's classification scheme nor were they instructed in filling it out. They were provided with examples and definitions to clarify each question.

Two methods are commonly used to establish rater agreement: percent agreement and Cohen's chance-corrected kappa statistic (Cohen, 1960). In general, percent agreement is the ratio of the number of times two raters agree divided by the total number of ratings performed. The kappa statistic estimates the proportion of agreement among raters after removing the proportion of agreement that would occur by chance. If the raters are in complete agreement, kappa equals 1. If there is no agreement among the raters (other than what would be expected by chance), kappa is less than or equal to 0.

To compute kappa, the PBAP first identified the "correct" answer for each question. Agreement was then computed based on the number of coders who agreed with the "correct" answer. Each coder read the case and supplied the information requested (e.g., age) or selected responses from predefined categories. TERCAP includes 60 questions; however, for each question where the coder was requested to check "all that apply," each answer category was treated as a separate question. Thus, for analysis purposes, 154 items were used in the final analysis. Kappa was computed as follows:

$$\kappa = \frac{P_A - P_C}{1 - P_C}$$

where:

P_A = proportion of units on which the raters agreed with the experts' designated correct answer.

P_C = the proportion of units for which agreement with the correct answer is expected by chance (1 ÷ number of response categories).

As an illustration, if 32 out of the 34 coders selected the "correct" answer for a particular question, the proportion of units on which the raters agreed with the experts' designated correct answer (P_A) would equal 0.94. If there were 13 possible response categories, the proportion of units for which agreement with the correct answer is expected by chance would equal 0.76. The kappa for that question is, therefore, 0.936.

The kappas for each question were added and divided by the number of questions to derive the mean or overall kappa for the TERCAP instrument. The kappas for each section of TERCAP were computed in the same manner. Section 1: Patient Profile, for example, included 16 questions. A kappa was computed for each of the 16 questions in that section. The mean of the 16 kappas represented the kappa for that section.

The desired level of inter-rater reliability that must be achieved for any given study has not been established clearly. Researchers generally think that values

TABLE 1.5 Overall and Section Inter-Rater Reliability of TERCAP by Coefficients of Agreement	
Sections by Title	Kappa
1. Patient Profile	0.80
2. Patient Outcome	0.67
3. Setting	0.78
4. Systems Issues	0.67
5. Health Care Team	0.70
6. Nurse Profile	0.78
7. Intentional Misconduct or Criminal Behavior	0.57
8. Safe Medication Administration	0.89
9. Documentation	0.74
10. Practice Breakdown Other Categories	0.68
Overall	0.75

greater than 0.75 or above may be taken to represent excellent agreement beyond chance, values below 0.40 may be taken to represent poor agreement beyond chance, and values between 0.40 and 0.75 are considered to represent fair to good agreement beyond chance (Capozzoli, McSweeney, & Sinha, 1999).

It is expected that the assessment of TERCAP will improve as groups make refinements to the instrument. As of the publication of this book, the coders, on average, agreed with the experts 97% of the time, and the overall inter-rater reliability achieved was 0.75 indicating excellent agreement between coders. The coefficients of agreement for each of the sections of TERCAP are shown in Table 1.5.

UTILITY

TERCAP is easy to administer. The electronic application is user friendly and includes links to the TERCAP coding protocol. Users in the pilot submitted TERCAPs based on discipline cases that had been completed in 2004 forward. The instructions required users to review the entire case file retrospectively, a process that can consume considerable time. The time to complete TERCAP took users between 20 minutes and 3 hours. The time factor was influenced by the familiarity of the user with the case and the ready availability of data. In future applications, investigators are likely to collect the information as a case progresses (e.g., using the instrument as an intake document that is attached to the case file). Once the case is resolved, the completed data will be entered into the electronic TERCAP for transmission to the NCSBN where the document will be stored for filing, retrieval, and analysis.

USING TERCAP—BOARDS OF NURSING

Boards of nursing are beginning to identify a variety of uses for TERCAP. TERCAP provides a consistent language to describe practice breakdown for board of nursing investigators, staff, and attorneys, and it guides the consistent and comprehensive collection of data. The categories of error and subcategories are being used to develop checklists for investigators to assist in data collection. TERCAP also provides a framework for case analysis that supports boards in their decision-making processes. Specific examples of the use of TERCAP by the North Dakota and Ohio Boards of Nursing are described in *Implications and Applications for State Boards of Nursing,* which can be found on the NCSBN's website at www.NCSBN.org.

PROCEDURES

ACCESS TO CASES

Members of the PBAP identified cases from their respective states that were completed within the last 60 months. They removed personal data from the cases prior to inclusion in the documents prepared for discussion and analysis.

DATA MANAGEMENT

Response categories created by the coders were identified as "not applicable," assigned a code (e.g., 999), and entered into the database when the response was not among a question's original response category. Invalid character values and invalid data that were either below or above expected ranges were transcribed exactly as they were written on the form. The only data that were modified were the dates transformed into their proper format of dd/mm/yyyy. The original hard copy data were retained to facilitate return to the original information. The NCSBN filed and stored the data for future retrieval.

DATA ANALYSIS

TO IMPROVE THE QUALITY OF THE DATA

The staff at NCSBN worked to improve the quality of data through several processes. To do this, they analyzed the differences between the given response categories, and they also analyzed respondents' answers. For example, a number of coders added categories such as "unknown" to some questions. These categories, if deemed necessary, were added to subsequent versions of the questionnaire.

TO ESTABLISH INTER-RATER RELIABILITY

As noted, inter-rater agreement and the kappa statistic were used to establish inter-rater reliability. The PBAP then reviewed prepared tables of the results by section and for the entire instrument.

The items on TERCAP will allow for descriptive statistics on the types of nursing practice breakdown that represent the major contributions to nursing practice breakdown at the state and national levels. The following correlation studies could be useful in understanding system, patient, and nurse characteristics associated with different levels of patient harm:

1. Correlation between the type of nursing practice breakdown and level of patient harm
2. Correlation between patient characteristics and types of practice breakdown and patient harm
3. Correlation between system sources of practice breakdown and types of practice breakdown
4. Correlation between nurse education and working patterns and type of practice breakdown

The electronic database will also provide an ongoing basis for assessing interventions at the state and national levels. In addition, the intake instrument (TERCAP) is sufficiently comprehensive to provide unanticipated data for analyzing specific types of practice breakdown prevalent in different types of health care institutions.

NCSBN will analyze and publish national data only. Individual state data will be published only with the expressed and written permission of the state board(s) of nursing. Individual states will be able to manage and analyze their data based on their needs. The findings from analysis of these data will provide evidence that has not been previously available to objectively advance the patient safety movement from the perspective of safe nursing practice. State boards of nursing will have the opportunity to conduct studies to determine whether specific state board educational interventions reduce certain classes of errors for nurses who have been reported. The collection of valid and reliable data and ongoing evaluation will continually reinforce and guide decision-making and strategy development.

SUMMARY

This practice breakdown research effort describes and classifies the characteristics of various nursing errors. The overall aim of the PBAP is far reaching. It is to promote patient safety by better understanding nursing practice breakdown and by improving the effectiveness of nursing regulation. The ultimate goal is to develop an interpretive guide for statistically analyzing data and writing a report that will include recommendations for nursing education and practice settings to reduce and prevent practice breakdown based on the actual reported incidents in each state.

These reports are expected to facilitate communication concerning the types of nursing errors and efforts at error prevention across states. Ultimately, the expectation is to transform a valuable, untapped, and unaggregated data set regarding actual errors into useful interpreted data that can provide concrete suggestions for reducing and preventing breakdown through education, system redesign, and enhanced individual and professional practice responsibility. These expectations are in keeping with the key principles that inform the work of boards of nursing in the United States and provide the needed evidence for a major change in the way nursing practice breakdown is viewed, understood, prevented, or decreased.

The adoption of a Web-based data collection instrument will advance the work of practice breakdown analysis. Data from TERCAP will be collected in the NCSBN national data center to allow for examination of the relationships between and among nurse demographics regarding category(s) of breakdown and system variables. The variability of patterns of errors can be compared between states and between types of systems, nurse characteristics, patient characteristics, working conditions, and system characteristics. Relationships between variables will be analyzed to identify new and more focused approaches to safe nursing practice.

The findings from analysis of these data will provide evidence that has not been previously available to objectively advance the patient safety movement from the perspective of safe nursing practice. State boards of nursing will have the opportunity to conduct studies to determine whether specific state board educational interventions reduce certain classes of errors for nurses who have been reported. The collection of valid and reliable data and ongoing evaluation will continually reinforce and guide decision-making that is reflective of clear problem identification, development of plans to address the problem, judgment of the feasibility of the plan, guidance regarding the implementation of the plan, and then provision of evidence from evaluation as a basis for any needed future revisions (rather than best guess decision-making). More information specific to the nature, scope, and causes of safety breaches will be identified using TERCAP.

We believe that this instrument and taxonomy of nursing practice can also be used by individual nurses in thinking about practice breakdown in their practices. It is also useful as an "upstream" data collection instrument in all health care delivery sites.

References

Aspden, P., Corrigan, J.M., Wolcott, J., Erickson, S.M. (Eds); Committee on Data Standards for Patient Safety; Institute of Medicine. (2004). *Patient safety: Achieving a new standard for care.* Washington, DC: The National Academies Press.

Aspden, P., Wolcott, J., Bootman, L., Cronenwett, L. (Eds); Committee on Identifying and Preventing Medication Errors, Institute of Medicine. (2006). *Preventing medication errors.* Washington, DC: The National Academies Press.

Benner, P., Hooper-Kyriakidis, P., & Stannard, D. (1999). *Clinical wisdom and interventions in critical care: Thinking-in-action approach.* Philadelphia: Saunders.

Benner, P., Sheets, V., Uris, P., Malloch, K., Schwed, K., & Jamison, D. (2002). Individual, practice, and system causes of errors in nursing: A taxonomy. *Journal of Nursing Administration, 32*(10), 509-523.

Benner, P., Sheets, V., Uris, P., Malloch, K., Schwed, K., Jamison, D., et al (2006). TERCAP: Creating a national database on nursing errors. *Harvard Health Policy Review, 7*(1), 48-63.

Benner, P., Sutphen, M., Leonard-Kahn, V., Day, L. (In press.) *Educating nurses: A call for radical transformation.* San Francisco: Jossey-Bass and Carnegie Foundation for the Advancement of Teaching.

Capozzoli, M., McSweeney, L., & Sinha, D. (1999). Beyond kappa: A review of inter-rater agreement measures. *The Canadian Journal of Statistics, 27*(1), 3-23.

Cohen, J. (1960). A coefficient of agreement for nominal scales. *Educational and Psychological Measurement,* 20, 37-46.

Committee on the Quality of Health Care in America, Institute of Medicine. (2001). *Crossing the quality chasm: A new health system for the 21st century.* Washington, DC: The National Academies Press.

Cooper, J.B., Gaba, D.M., Liang, B., Woods, D., & Blum, L.N. (2000). The National Patient Safety Foundation Agenda for Research and Development in Patient Safety. *Medscape General Medicine, 2*(3), E38.

Cronenwett, L., Sherwood, G., Barnsteiner, J., Disch, J., Johnson, J., Mitchell, P., et al (2007). Quality and safety education for nurses. *Nursing Outlook, 55*(3), 122-131.

Gawande, A. (2007). Annals of Medicine: The Checklist. If something so simple can transform intensive care, what else can it do? *The New Yorker,* December 10, 2007.

Greiner, A.C., Knebel E. (Eds.); Committee on the Health Professions Education Summit, Institute of Medicine. (2003). *Health professions education: A bridge to quality.* Washington, DC: The National Academies Press.

Kohn, L.T., Corrigan, J.M., & Donaldson, M.S. (Eds); Committee on Quality of Health Care in America, Institute of Medicine. (2000). *To err is human: Building a safer health system.* Washington, DC: The National Academies Press.

Leape, L.L., Lawthers, A.G., Brennan, T.A., & Johnson, W.G. (1993). Preventing medical injury. *Quality Review Bulletin, 19*(5), 144-149.

Liang, B.A. (2006). Addressing the nursing work environment to promote nursing safety. *Nursing Forum,* 42(1), 20-30.

MacIntyre, A. (1984). *After virtue: A study in moral theory* (2nd ed.). Indianapolis: University of Notre Dame Press.

Marx, D. (2001). *Patient safety and the "just culture": A primer for health care executives.* New York: Columbia University Press.

National Patient Safety Foundation. (1999). *Focus on patient safety.* Available online at www.npsf.org. Retrieved November 17, 2008.

Page, A. (Ed.); Committee on the Work Environment for Nurses and Patient Safety, Institute of Medicine. *Keeping patients safe: Transforming the work environment of nurses.* (2004). Washington, DC: The National Academies Press.

Pope, B.B., Rodzen, L., & Spross, G. (2008). Raising the SBAR: How better communication improves patient outcomes. *Nursing, 38*(3):41-43.

Reason, J. (1990). *Human error.* Cambridge: Cambridge University Press.

Reason, J. (1997). *Managing the risks of organizational accidents.* Burlington, VT: Ashgate Publications.

Stone, P.W., Mooney-Kane, C., Larson, E.L., Horan, T., Glance, L.G., Zwanziger, J., et al. (2007). Nurse working conditions and patient safety outcomes. *Medical Care, 45*(6), 571-578.

Sullivan, W. (2004). *Work and integrity: The crisis and promise of professionalism in America* (2nd ed.) San Francisco: Jossey-Bass.

Sullivan, W. (2005). Challenges to professionalism: Work integrity and the call to renew and strengthen the social contract of the professions. *American Journal of Critical Care, 14*(1), 78-80, 84.

Vincent, C. (2003). Understanding and responding to adverse events. *New England Journal of Medicine, 348*(11), 1051-1056.

Vincent, C., Taylor-Adams, S., & Stanhope, N. (1998). Framework for analysing risk and safety in clinical medicine. *BMJ*, *316*(7138), 1154-1157.

Wachter, R.M. (2008). *Understanding patient safety*. New York: McGraw Hill Medical.

Wachter, R.M., & Shojania, K.G. (2004). *Internal bleeding: The truth behind America's terrifying epidemic of medical mistakes*. New York: Rugged Land.

Weick, K.E., & Sutcliff, K.M. (2001). *Managing the unexpected: Assuring high performance in an age of complexity*. San Francisco: Jossey-Bass.

Woods, P.J. (2004). *Integrating evidence-based nursing practice into education, research and patient care*. Paper presented at the 2004 Quality Colloquium, Harvard University, Cambridge, MA.

Wu, A.W. (2000). Medical error: The second victim. *Western Journal of Medicine*, *172*(6), 358-359.

Wu, A.W., Folkman, S., McPhee, S.J., & Lo, B. (1991). Do house officers learn from their mistakes? *Journal of the American Medical Association*, *265*(16), 2089-2094.

2

Practice Breakdown: Medication Administration

Lisa Emrich

Chapter Outline

Ensuring the safe administration of medications within the health care system is complex and requires a health care professional's attention to multiple factors during the process. No one professional can prevent all medication errors. The nurse is at the sharp end of delivery of medications that may have started out wrong in the physician's order, in the drug packaging, in the pharmacy, or in labeling and packaging similarities. The professional who is attentive to these multiple factors increases the chances for safe medication administration. In order to reliably and safely administer medications, the nurse needs to determine the patient's condition and/or stability, the actions and side effects of the medication to be administered, the patient's current medications, the patient's environment, and the activities that other health care professionals are carrying out on behalf of the patient. Conscious patients should be enlisted to assist with safe administration of medication by clearly identifying themselves to the nurse and being informed of their medications taken at home and in the hospital.

Adverse medication effects can occur even under optimal conditions. A medication combined with other medications, substances, and/or the patient's physiology has the potential to create life-threatening reactions within the patient, causing temporary or permanent harm to the patient. Computerized information programs on drug interactions, solubility, safe routes, dosages, and complications are an indispensable aid in avoiding delivery of a contraindicated drug to a patient. The nurse must learn to use these systems, and hospitals need to ensure their accessibility to all members of the health care team.

Considerable effort is devoted to mastering the requisite knowledge related to finding the best information on the actions and synergistic effects of medications, incompatibilities, and the ways in which groups and individual patients respond to specific medications. This effort is well spent and essential, because of the array of potential adverse reactions that may occur. Each individual patient's responses need to be evaluated to determine whether the response to the administered medications is within the expected range or if the patient is having adverse reactions.

Nurses who are knowledgeable about patients' illnesses and medications are able to provide competent care as they are alert to information sources about the known or expected side effects, medication contraindications, and incompatibilities. Clearly, nurses are well positioned as the patient's last line of defense to protect patients from unsafe medication administration by using all the available resources pertaining to the particular patient and medication, double-checking all aspects of medication appropriateness in terms of correct dosage, route of administration, timing, purpose, and whether this is the correct patient (Page, 2004).

Identified points within the processing of medications that are particularly vulnerable to practice breakdown noted above include medication prescribing or ordering, dispensing, and administration (Williams, 2004). Nurses' work takes place primarily at the health care system-to-patient interface, and medication administration is a traditional nursing role within this context. The Institute of Medicine (IOM) discussed these types of practice breakdown as "errors" in its report *To Err Is Human* (Kohn et al., 2000), in which it described latent errors as those being removed from the direct control of the operator (or in this case the nurse) and include as poor design and poor management decisions or policies. The IOM report describes an active error as an action of the frontline operator in which the results are immediately known. For example, a nurse may convert a latent error to an active error by not recognizing that a medication with a name similar to ibuprofen was erroneously dispensed by a pharmacy. As a result, a nurse may accidentally administer bupropion (Wellbutrin) to the patient instead of ibuprofen.

Investigators discussed possible causes leading to medication errors and nurse involvement:

> ...medication errors, an activity directly involving nursing care, have been the subject of many of the studies on error. Within this research focus, studies have typically analyzed errors associated with the order and administration of medications. All too common and preventable are errors such as inappropriate dosage, overlooked known allergies, and wrong drug or route of administration. Such errors often stem from a confluence of factors including environmental distractions, miscommunications, and drug-labeling problems (Maddox, Wakefield, & Bull, 2001, p. 10).

Distractions in the form of noise, interruptions, multitasking, and work over-load seriously hamper the nurse's ability to administer medications safely. Health professionals who report their perceptions of why errors occur frequently cite interruptions and distractions (Ely et al., 1995; Gladstone, 1995). Relying on memory is dangerous, and the nurse, like all members of the health care team, needs to avoid reliance on memory related to drug actions, dosages, inter-actions, and contraindications. The nurse must evaluate and double-check for errors in the medication order, in misspelled or unclear orders, the manner in which the order was transcribed, and the route by which the medication was dis-pensed. Nurses often identify and correct a significant number of errors com-mitted by other health care professionals (Page, 2004) before the error reaches the patient. However, no health care team member is ever exempt from unin-tended medication error.

When the nurse does not check appropriate resources, lacks knowledge about particular patient risks, or for any reason tries to cover up a medication error, this results in the employer's corrective actions and the potential license sanc-tions of the nurse's regulatory board, when such sanctions are warranted.

Regardless of the outcomes of such investigations, these institutional and reg-ulatory reviews are opportunities to examine and evaluate the factors pertaining to the error and to learn more about the role of the various individuals and sys-tems in the error. In this regard, an effective evaluation means that a practice breakdown scenario undergoes review as one system with many subsystems. An open and just culture that does not focus on blame or shame but rather on improving patient quality and patient safety is essential for maximum disclo-sure and review of all medication errors. A systematic review of relevant informa-tion can lead to the creation of methodologic comparisons of the system and of the health care team's and the individuals' contributions to the ultimate end point of an error in the administration of medication. These elements can be seen within the context of other systems and other individuals' behavior, noting the system's and the nurse's strengths and weaknesses. Learning from this anal-ysis can be shared with the institutions and with health care regulators and edu-cators. Highly reliable complex systems are alert to potential breakdowns and errors, and respond by cross-checking one another's performance, avoiding reli-ance on memory, and constantly analyzing near-misses as well as errors in order to continuously improve reliability and safety (Weick & Sutcliff, 2001).

Many state and federal agencies and organizations have created methods to openly review and evaluate medication errors to improve patient safety. As noted, this is accomplished by identifying, reducing, and ultimately eliminating the opportunities for error at the multiple points in the system of ordering and administering medications (Agency for Healthcare Research and Quality, 2008; Institute of Safe Medication Practices, 2008; The Joint Commis-sion, 2008). For example, the Institute of Safe Medication Practices (ISMP) has prepared a list of medications that subject patients to heightened risk when the medications are erroneously administered (2008). Health care institutions can establish policies and procedures concerning these specific medications in response to well-established heightened risks of particular medications. Further, agencies have also worked to identify and eliminate the use of dangerous abbreviations to decrease the risk for errors associated with misinterpretation of medication prescriptions and orders (Agency for Healthcare Research and Quality, 2008; ISMP, 2008; *Ohioans First*, 2004, 2009; The Joint Commission, 2008). Institutional failure to attend to these interventions (i.e., automatic alerts to heightened risk medications, use of dangerous abbreviations, lack of automated warnings of drug contraindications and dangerous interactions) place the nurse at unnecessary increased risk for making medication errors, especially in highly pressured work environments.

The Joint Commission's National Patient Safety Goals (2008) have called for the removal of concentrated electrolytes from clinical units, thus decreasing another opportunity for erroneous administration. For example, potentially lethal concentrations of potassium chloride are no longer stored in patient's medications or on the patient care unit.

When nurses' actions result in a primary medication error, the error is seldom due to the nurse's lack of knowledge about the mechanics of medication administration. Rather, the error tends to be due to the nurse's knowledge deficit about the medication and its effect on the patient's clinical situation. The nurse's inability to recall specific knowledge that should be applied at the time the medication is being administered may also lead to the nurse's commission of a primary error. With the proliferation of pharmaceuticals, nurses should be discouraged from relying on recall alone, although they are responsible for knowing the major classes and actions of pharmaceuticals. Therefore the questions most pertinent to ask when reviewing the nurse's activities in each error scenario are:

- What information should the nurse have checked but did not?
- What general knowledge about pharmaceutical classes and actions of drugs was missing?
- Did the nurse properly research and apply the knowledge he/she checked in relation to the medication being administered?
- What knowledge or pharmaceutical references and medication safety cross-checks did the nurse not have access to that, if the resource had been available at the time he/she administered the medication, would have changed the nurse's actions?

As automated medication systems of delivery are added, new types of errors are likely to develop (Reason, 1990).

For the State Board of Nursing an important question is: What is the regulatory culpability of a nurse concerning the absence of his/her knowledge in general about the safe administration of medication, and what knowledge about and availability or actual use of the relevant pharmaceutical reference sources contributed to the error? In its recent report, *Keeping Patients Safe: Transforming the Work Environment for Nurses* (Page, 2004), the IOM recommended that the NCSBN work with constituent boards to create a system of identifying and differentiating nurses' acts of human error from those of willful misconduct.

Regardless of its root cause, be it a system issue or individual accountability, the resulting medication error jeopardizes patients' health and well-being, and nurses and other members of the health care team do not usually willfully set out to harm patients. The activities and behaviors of nurses involved in medication errors are explored at the regulatory level when an error greatly harms the patient or goes beyond the usual acts of human error. Both the health care delivery site and the regulatory boards are responsible for examining the complexity and dynamics of the system, the health care community, and nurse and patient variables that contributed to the error. In the TERCAP® instrument, all of these areas are addressed. The database provided by this tool will provide additional information about heightened-risk medication, as well as heightened risks for medication errors associated with the work environment, the collaborative and communication efficacy of the organization, the effective, collaborative functioning of the health care team, and patient conditions such as cognitive impairment that lead to higher risks for medication errors.

TERCAP provides a framework to collect, analyze, and disseminate the factors that comprise and contribute to medication administration errors by accurately categorizing the behavior of nurses and others, and thoughts about their activities at the time of the error. In addition, TERCAP identifies factors that are external to and at the perimeter of the involved nurse's professional control, but may have contributed to the nursing practice breakdown, resulting in a medication error. It is important that these factors be identified and discussed in the context of the health care environment, the nurse-patient situation, and the resulting error, so that the learning that occurs can be applied to subsequent nurse-patient situations and similar errors may be prevented.

CASE ANALYSES

Errors that involve nurses' administration of medications are examined in this section and discussed in conjunction with the use of TERCAP. Here scenarios are presented about errors that involve the administration of medications by nurses. Reviews follow these descriptions with explanations as to the ways in which various behaviors, activities, and pertinent clinical information contained within each scenario may be captured by TERCAP.

HISTORICAL CASE STUDY #1: The Chemotherapy Protocol

PRACTICE BREAKDOWN IN MEDICATION ADMINISTRATION

HISTORY

Mr. Michael Neal, a young man diagnosed as having cancer, was being treated with a chemotherapeutic agent in accordance with a highly strict research protocol. The protocol involved intravenously infusing Mr. Neal through his central venous line with twice the standard dose of the chemotherapeutic agent over a

24-hour period. The infusion was repeated once every 7 days. The nursing staff used an infusion pump to regulate the patient's chemotherapy infusion.

Ms. Jane Jones, a certified oncology nurse, held a senior rank within the institution's clinical ladder and served as a resource for other clinical staff. She initiated and discontinued Mr. Neal's chemotherapy infusion during a specific week (as specified in the protocol). However, at the end of the 24-hour infusion period, Nurse Jones saw that 10 to 20 mL of the infusion remained in the bag. Nurse Jones *bolused* Mr. Neal with this remaining amount of the chemotherapeutic agent in accordance with what Nurse Jones identified as standard procedure regarding left-over amounts of chemotherapeutic agents. Nurse Jones did not document that she had bolused the 10 to 20 mL of the remaining agent, nor did she inform Mr. Neal's attending physician of the bolused remaining amount.

The following week Ms. Jones again initiated and discontinued Mr. Neal's chemotherapy infusion. However, by the end of the 24-hour infusion period, only half of the infusion had been administered, leaving approximately 50 to 60 mL of the chemotherapeutic agent in the infusion bag. Ms. Jones again bolused the remaining 50 to 60 mL of medication.

Nurse Jones did not report a possible infusion pump malfunction to the facility's bioengineering department. Nor did anyone else report this possibility. Further, no information in the documentation indicated that other health care professionals were notified during the tenure of Nurse Jones's care that the infusion was falling behind.

Two days after the treatment, Mr. Neal reported swelling and other symptoms to his physician. Mr. Neal was later diagnosed with septic shock, liver disease progression, and stomatitis. Nurse Jones, on learning of Mr. Neal's symptoms, informed the attending physician of her previous administration of the two boluses of the chemotherapeutic agent. It was at this time that she made a late entry in Mr. Neal's record concerning the boluses of medication.

ANALYSIS

This brief scenario reveals much information about the patient situation and Nurse Jones's behaviors and activities. She used knowledge from her past clinical experience and situations but inappropriately applied the knowledge to the current patient circumstance. It appears that Nurse Jones's actions were task oriented and did not reveal the ongoing mindfulness necessary to provide safe nursing care. She did not take into account that the chemotherapy was being administered under a strict research protocol with a much higher than usual level of chemotherapy. It was not apparent that Nurse Jones considered a bolus of the concentration of the chemotherapeutic agent she administered to be highly toxic to Mr. Neal because she had carried out this same practice with much lower concentrations of chemotherapy in the past.

The attending physician was not notified in a timely manner of Nurse Jones' deviation from the prescribed protocol, either directly by her or indirectly through her documentation. The physician was unaware of the change in dosage and therefore did not alter any procedure relative to Mr. Neal's initial chemotherapy underdose and subsequent overdose. In this regard, opportunity was lost for immediate rescue of the patient from the medication's toxic effects.

No mention was noted of the care other nurses provided preceding Nurse Jones' discontinuing the infusion. However, it would appear that no one noticed that the infusion had fallen behind. Although there could have been a miscalculation of the infusion rate, there was also a possibility that the infusion pump had malfunctioned. The infusion pump was not removed, and this uncorrected situation provided the possibility for further error.

The TERCAP instrument includes a category and subcategories that capture the preceding nursing activities and other factors that may contribute to a breakdown in nursing practice and a resulting medication error. This TERCAP section, Safe Medication Administration, captures information about medication administration and provides space to document what did and did not occur within the activities designated as medication preparation and administration.

In this case, the medication ordered was administered, and it was administered via the correct intravenous route. However, the dose that was infused differed from the dose that was ordered. TERCAP asks for the type of medication error. In this instance, improper dose/quantity and incorrect administration technique are the types of medication errors that occurred.

In this scenario, Nurse Jones did not follow the procedure/protocol as she administered an incorrect dose/quantity of the medication. Further, the situation was additionally compromised by the failure or malfunction of the pump. Because the error also involved the medication infusion rate, the applicable factors may include a miscalculation of dosage or infusion rate, which would also be captured under the category of performance deficit.

After Nurse Jones discovered that the patient did not receive the full dose of the chemotherapy, she unfortunately gave the patient the remaining amount that was left in the bag as a result pump malfunction. This was a new "high dose chemotherapy regime," and therefore, should not have been administered all at once. The unit nurses had, in the past, given varying amounts of remaining chemotherapeutic agents without obvious patient harm when the chemotherapy dosages were lower. Now that the chemotherapy dosages were so much higher, giving remaining amounts all at once became a lethal, unexamined, and unsanctioned practice. There had been little or no safety orientation and training for the new higher concentration of chemotherapeutic agents. There was no crosschecking of physician and nurse informal practices and no communication about them, so physicians were unaware that nurses were routinely bolusing in remainders of chemotherapy left after 24-hour infusions. Here it is important to note that, based on her documented clinical expertise, the nurse had knowledge of, but did not think about, the risks of the concentrated medication bolus.

The causes, nurse's knowledge and performance deficit, the machine malfunction, and inadequate orientation and training for the new higher doses of chemotherapy all influenced this tragic error that caused the patient's death. The nurse's delayed discussion with Mr. Neal's physician concerning the initial underdosing or break in the research protocol and the inaction by anyone to notify bioengineering to examine the functioning of the infusion pump or to remove it from the patient care area were related to a culture of low expectations for equipment performance, and a well-established but an unexamined, unsafe informal routine of bolusing in remainders of IV chemotherapy at the end of 24 hours, prior to hanging a new IV of chemotherapy. Had Nurse Jones been informed about the risks of the newer higher concentrations of chemotherapy in a timely update or inservice education, this chain of unfortunate mishaps could have been avoided. The fact that she did not inform the physician earlier about bolusing in the additional chemotherapy was caused by her lack of understanding of the consequences of the higher dosage of chemotherapy, and using an unexamined and unsafe informal practice.

HISTORICAL CASE STUDY #2: A Groupthink Error

PRACTICE BREAKDOWN IN MEDICATION ADMINISTRATION

HISTORY

An attending physician ordered the administration of 50,000 units/kg of penicillin G/benzathine intramuscularly to a full-term infant, Baby Sandy. Ms. Erin Smith, a registered nurse assigned to care for the infant, sent the order to the pharmacy and subsequently received two syringes of penicillin G/benzathine from the pharmacy.

The two syringes contained a total medication volume of 2.5 mL. The unit's policy concerning infant intramuscular injections allowed for a maximum medication volume of 0.5 mL per injection. After receiving the two syringes of medication, Nurse Smith commented briefly to her unit colleagues about the number of times she would be required to stick the infant. She then began her other unit activities before returning to administer the injections to Baby Sandy.

On Nurse Smith's return to attend to Baby Sandy, Nurse Smith noted that Ms. Marcy Davis, the unit's nurse practitioner, and Ms. Margo Johnson, a registered nurse also working in the unit that day, were researching information about penicillin and the injections that were to be administered to Baby Sandy. Their joint goal was to decrease or eliminate the need for Baby Sandy to receive multiple intramuscular injections.

Before filling and dispensing Baby Sandy's penicillin G/benzathine, the hospital pharmacist called the nursing unit to obtain the infant's weight. However, unknown to Nurse Smith, Nurse Davis, and Nurse Johnson, the pharmacist misinterpreted the order. He prepared 500,000 units of the penicillin per kg of the infant's weight instead of the ordered 50,000 units per kg.

The pharmacist did correctly note that penicillin G/benzathine was a viscous solution and therefore labeled the two syringes of penicillin G/benzathine as "IM USE ONLY" before dispensing the penicillin G/benzathine to the nursing unit.

While Nurse Smith was attending to her other nursing activities, Nurse Johnson consulted with Nurse Davis to see if the medication could be administered intravenously, thus negating the need for injecting the baby through multiple intramuscular injections.

Nurse Davis and Nurse Johnson consulted two drug references for "penicillin G" in one reference and "penicillin G potassium/penicillin G sodium" in another. Both of the references for these medications indicated that the penicillin could be administered intravenously. Nurse Davis informed Nurse Smith that both Nurse Davis and Nurse Johnson would administer the penicillin to the infant.

Nurse Davis changed the physician's order for the route of the penicillin administration from intramuscular to intravenous. Nurse Johnson started the infant's IV and intravenously administered the penicillin G/benzathine to the infant. Baby Sandy expired.

ANALYSIS

This was a tragic and certainly unintended human error starting in the pharmacy and ending with the nurses in the neonatal ICU. Staying curious and being concerned about unusual amounts and routes of administration are habits of the mind that are needed by all members of the health care team. Errors do not start out to be errors, and in this case the error was neither prevented nor understood until after the medication was administered to the infant.

The medication ordered was indeed the medication administered and would be documented on TERCAP in the section identified under Safe Medication Administration. However, the dose administered was 10 times greater than the dose that was ordered, and the route by which the medication was administered was inappropriate for the viscous medication. Therefore, in responding to TERCAP, the types of medication error one would enter are improper dose/quantity and incorrect route.

Two primary errors occurred in this case. One was by the pharmacist who misread the physician order and dispensed the wrong dose of the medication, and one by Nurse Davis who gave the order for the medication to be administered intravenously. In this instance, the major factors that contributed to the medication error would be coded as "performance (human) deficit" related to the pharmacist's dispensing error and as "knowledge deficit" related to the nurse practitioner's mistaken belief that the medication could be safely administered intravenously. The actions of these two health care professionals certainly contributed to the practice breakdown.

Nurse Johnson, however, by not recognizing either of the other professionals' errors, perpetuated the error sequence by administering the medication. One important question that this case presents is: To what extent is Nurse Johnson culpable as the nurse who administered the penicillin? It is also important to review and discuss these nurses' decision points within this scenario.

DECISION POINTS WITHIN THE SCENARIO

The first decision point occurred at the time the nurses on the unit received the dispensed medication. All three of the nurses were in agreement that the volume of medication that was to be injected was excessive and recognized/cited the unit's policy concerning the maximum amount of intramuscular injectate for infants. Despite their collective knowledge that the volume dispensed was five times the acceptable injection volume, the problem-solving attention of these nurses was directed to avoiding the multiple injections rather than questioning the reasons the volume was excessive. This is a good example of a human tendency to identify and fixate on the wrong problem, excessive volume, rather than questioning the accuracy of this amount of volume. A good maxim for medication administration is that packaging is usually congruent with the proper dosage level. When this maxim is violated, the nurse should question the accuracy of the dose. Had the nurses included the pharmacist and prescribing physician in this early discussion, the dispensing decision may have been revealed.

The second decision point concerned the exclusion of Nurse Smith, the infant's primary care nurse, from the medication administration scenario. In this instance, the extent of Nurse Smith's involvement in averting the error cannot be determined.

The third decision point concerned Nurse Practitioner Davis, and Nurse Johnson's consultation of the drug references. The nurses did not identify penicillin G/benzathine specifically in the drug reference, and thus their actions were based on incomplete information. Further, Nurse Practitioner Davis and Nurse Johnson did not observe the "IM USE ONLY" label on the dispensed syringes of penicillin. This unintended concentration of errors provides an important cautionary tale. The effects of the tragic loss of the newborn baby's life on the parents and on the nurses cannot be underestimated. This costly error needs to be publicized within the institution as a crucial learning point so that such an incident will be less likely in the future.

HISTORICAL CASE STUDIES #3 AND #4: The Right Medication, The Wrong Route

TWO SCENARIOS OF PRACTICE BREAKDOWN IN MEDICATION ADMINISTRATION

ADMINISTRATION

The following two scenarios each involved a nurse who administered medication inappropriately. Although the scenarios have some similarities, their differences are quite distinct.

HISTORICAL CASE STUDY #3

Ms. Emily Mugford was a middle-aged woman who was severely mentally and developmentally delayed. She was admitted to a hospital's medical-surgical unit for complaints of dyspnea, weakness, and anorexia. Her physician ordered an abdominal CT scan.

Ms. Sarah Lynn, a relatively new associate degree graduate, had been working as a registered nurse for approximately 9 months and was in her second week of orientation in her new staff nurse position on the medical-surgical unit of the hospital. She had held a part-time clinic position before starting her current, full-time job and was working 7:00 AM to 7:00 PM on the day that Ms. Mugford was to have her abdominal CT scan. Nurse Lynn had previously been assigned five patients during a shift. However, on the day of the incident she had been assigned 10 patients.

Nurse Lynn and the team leader, Ms. Connie Rand, who was also Nurse Lynn's preceptor, were in the unit's medication room. Mr. Sidney Banner, identified as a member of the radiology department, approached them and asked for a syringe. Nurse Lynn initially handed Mr. Banner a 3 mL syringe. Mr. Banner stated that he needed "something bigger." Nurse Lynn then handed Mr. Banner a 20 mL syringe and asked "if it would do." Mr. Banner took the syringe and left the room. Before approaching Nurse Lynn and Nurse Rand in the medication room, Mr. Banner had arrived on the medical-surgical unit with a paper cup filled with oral contrast. He took the cup of contrast into Ms. Mugford's room, set it on the bedside table, and after observing that a 60 mL syringe was at the bedside for use in feeding Ms. Mugford, he went to the nurses' station to retrieve another syringe to administer the oral contrast. Mr. Banner received the syringe from Nurse Lynn, returned to Ms. Mugford's room, left the contrast and the syringe at her bedside, returned again to the nurses' station, and informed Nurse Lynn and Nurse Rand that he did not have time to administer the contrast. He said that he had left the contrast in the room, and asked if either Nurse Lynn or Nurse Rand could administer it.

Nurse Lynn told Nurse Rand that she would go to Ms. Mugford's room to administer the contrast. On entering Ms. Mugford's room, Nurse Lynn found the paper cup of contrast sitting on the over-bed table. The syringe that Nurse Lynn had previously given Mr. Banner was filled with contrast and was positioned by the cup on the table. According to Nurse Lynn, she picked up the syringe, removed a needle from her pocket, placed the needle on the syringe, and proceeded to intravenously administer the contrast to Ms. Mugford.

Ms. Mugford immediately went into respiratory distress and cardiopulmonary arrest. No one had witnessed Nurse Lynn's administration of the contrast to Ms. Mugford, and the information was not disclosed to anyone who responded to Nurse Lynn's request for assistance when Ms. Mugford's condition deteriorated rapidly. A resuscitation team was not called because of the presence of a "do not resuscitate" order in Ms. Mugford's medical record.

Nurse Lynn stated that her initial thought as to the cause of the change in Ms. Mugford's condition was that she was having an allergic reaction to the contrast. It was not until later in the afternoon, while speaking about the incident with another nurse that Nurse Lynn began to give thought to her intravenous administration of the contrast as being an erroneous act. Nurse Lynn then spoke with the Director of Nursing about the incident at which time Nurse Lynn disclosed her actions.

Further interviews with Nurse Lynn and others revealed additional information about the events that led to the incident. Nurse Rand was Nurse Lynn's nursing school co-graduate, and had been working in another department of the hospital for about 2 months prior to transferring to the medical-surgical unit. This was the first time that Nurse Rand had served as a preceptor.

Mr. Banner was the secretary/receptionist for the radiology department. He noted that an x-ray technician had mixed Ms. Mugford's oral contrast in anticipation of the CT scan and gave it to Mr. Banner to take to Ms. Mugford, as was customary practice for the radiology department. A review of the physician's order for the CT scan in Ms. Mugford's chart did not reveal an order for contrast to be administered in conjunction with the examination.

On Nurse Lynn's initial employment at the hospital, her former employer and her nursing school instructors provided very positive recommendations on her behalf. Nurse Lynn described her orientation at the hospital as "following another nurse for a day and being assigned three patients the second day," noting that she had never heard the terms "preceptor" or "team leader," and that no one had ever accompanied her when she was providing care to patients. Nurse Lynn stated that the unit manager had met with her, told her "some things," and had instructed her to find somebody if she experienced trouble. However, information indicates that prior to the incident, Nurse Lynn had met with her unit manager at which time Nurse Lynn reviewed and signed a document indicating that her orientation was going well. When specifically asked about the incident and her actions, Nurse Lynn stated that there was no label on the cup that contained the contrast, and she assumed that it was to be administered by IV push because it was her understanding that only registered nurses administered IV push medications and licensed practical nurses "did everything else." Nurse Lynn stated she had not previously administered any intravenous medications. Although she stated she had been provided a "skills checklist" that was being checked off, she was not able to produce the list after the incident.

Nurse Lynn was terminated from her position at the hospital and returned to work at the clinic. The physician there reported that Nurse Lynn was "quite green and...had a lot to learn." However, the physician thought Nurse Lynn worked well at the clinic and attributed Nurse Lynn's problems to "lack of experience and training."

HISTORICAL CASE STUDY #4

Another scenario concerned a registered nurse who had been working as a nurse for 4 months. Ms. Kathryn Murphy, a nurse with a bachelor's degree, successfully completed her 6- to 8-week preceptee orientation 1 month prior to the incident. Nurse Murphy worked in the hospital's float pool on a day and night rotation.

She alerted a physician about her patient, Mr. Steve Shapiro, whose serum potassium level was 2.5 mEq/dL. Not long after the notification, Nurse Murphy stated that Mr. Shapiro's attending physician called in response to the reported hypokalemia and provided Nurse Murphy with a telephone order to "give 40 mEq KCl bolus." Nurse Murphy stated that she repeated the order to the physician and the physician confirmed "that's right." However, instead of first writing the telephone order in the patient's record, Nurse Murphy withdrew the KCl from the unit's stock medication system, measured 40 mEq of KCl, and administered the medication by IV push via Mr. Shapiro's Groshong catheter.

Mr. Shapiro began convulsing at which time the unit charge nurse came to the bedside. Nurse Murphy immediately informed the charge nurse "I just gave the KCl IV push." The charge nurse responded "oh my God, you didn't," which is when Nurse Murphy realized she had made a grave mistake. Nurse Murphy became visibly upset and was taken to an anteroom.

REVIEW OF PROCEDURE FOLLOWED

The float pool nurse manager came to speak with Nurse Murphy and brought Nurse Murphy the patient's chart for her to write the KCl telephone order that she received from the physician. A subsequent review of the chart with entries during that time period revealed that in the interim, the physician, who had been summoned to the patient's bedside, had already written his order as "KCl 40 mEq IVPB × 1 over 4 hours." Nurse Murphy then wrote the order she received from the physician, as "add KCL 40 mEq to MIV." In addition, Nurse Murphy made an entry in the nurse notes as follows: "Received T.O. from Dr. Smith to add KCl 40 mEq to MIV and to give a bolus of 40 mEq of KCl. KCl 40 mEq bolus given IV . . . Dr. called to room."

The physician's progress note stated that he was called to see the patient because the patient was in ventricular fibrillation and he had no electrical cardiac activity. The patient's record also included a "do not resuscitate" code status.

When Nurse Murphy was questioned about the error, she stated that she thought it occurred because she followed the physician's orders and that she did not know that potassium chloride IV push was contraindicated. Nurse Murphy resigned her position at the hospital and subsequently began work at another facility on the day shift. She did not disclose the medication error to the new employer, and at the time of this error there were no State Board of Nursing databases that tracked individual nurses' errors before they started a new job (see Chapter 10). Nurse Murphy has not incurred further practice problems, her evaluations have been positive, and she states she carries a drug reference book with her at all times.

COMPARATIVE ANALYSIS

In these two cases, both nurses were relatively inexperienced, which contributed considerably to the medication errors that occurred. Had Nurse Lynn relied on the basic standard of verifying medication orders, verifying the medication, and ensuring aseptic technique, she would not have administered the oral contrast intravenously. A more serious basic question of deep learning or formation in nursing school about sterile and nonsterile fields underlies these acts. The lack of sterility of the contrast medium, and the viscosity and opaqueness of the solution, should have been have been sufficiently salient to Nurse Lynn to deter her automated or routinized, action without thought. No human being, regardless of experience, is immune to lapses of thoughtfulness; however, professional formation and overtraining of habits of thoughts and actions in some essential errors should create an additional layer of protection to the actions of any well-prepared professional, regardless of the field. Each field has its own central habits and tenets, and sense of salience, and habits around "sterile, dirty, and clean fields" are among the basic habits of thought and action in nursing. Nurse Lynn's response about acting on role descriptions of what registered nurses (RNs) do and what licensed vocational nurses (LVNs) do, reveals a "job description" understanding of the RN role and a lack of grasp of the professional accountability for knowledge and judgment of both levels of nursing practice.

Further, information suggests that Nurse Lynn's orientation was not well designed and that Nurse Rand, because of her own inexperience, was an inappropriate choice for Nurse Lynn's preceptor. However, Nurse Rand later testified that she felt competent to be a preceptor.

The question remains that if Nurse Lynn's absence of appropriate insight, knowledge, and judgment had been detected during the first week of her orientation, her practice would likely have been more tightly monitored and documented than it was. These orientation concerns would be important to document by the state board investigator using TERCAP.

Nurse Murphy was conscientious about her responsibilities but was inexperienced as a staff nurse. She had successfully completed her orientation period, and documentation was available to attest to this action. She asserted good judgment in promptly reporting Mr. Shapiro's hypokalemia to the physician but did not possess adequate knowledge of the risks of intravenous potassium before she administered this medication. The nurse's knowledge deficit was compounded by the availability of the concentrated electrolyte through the unit's automated dispensing system. It is noteworthy that this particular error has since been rendered almost impossible to make because concentrated electrolytes are no longer stored on patient care units.

Nurse Murphy was accurate and responsible in reporting all of her actions to the charge nurse at the time of the incident and realized, with the charge nurse's response, that her actions were erroneous. However, Nurse Murphy affirmatively stated that she was following the physician's verbal order to give the "KCl bolus," which was different from the order the physician wrote in the patient's record immediately after being called to the patient's bedside.

It is speculative that the physician abbreviated the telephone order that was given to Nurse Murphy, possibly expecting her to further interpret the order. However, no information is available that this was confirmed by the state board case investigator. If, indeed, this "shorthand" communication was the medium of communication, it illustrates the ways in which communication or miscommunication often plays an active role in medication errors. It is likely that the physician thought of the slower administration of KCl as a boost or "bolus," although this is **not** the common use of the term "bolus" for nurses.

The NCSBN's Model Administrative Rules (2004) delineate the general requirements of states' nurse practice acts. These include the standard that each registered nurse clarify orders when needed, especially "phone orders" (first by clarifying on the phone and second by looking up the safety and reasonableness of the order). Currently undergraduate nurses have little experience in phoning a doctor for a provider order (Benner, Sutphen, Leonard, & Day, in press). This incident illustrates the need for instruction and at least simulated practice in obtaining emergency medication for a rapidly changing or dangerous patient condition. From Ms. Murphy's perspective, she very well understood the physician's order to give the "KCl bolus," and erroneously she considered *this* to be sufficient warrant for her actions with no additional cross-checking of her colleague's order.

In Reason's (1991) theory, the holes in the Swiss cheese lined up perfectly to allow this tragic error to occur. Concentrated vials of KCl were then readily available on the patient care unit; the physician was unclear about the nursing meaning or interpretation of the word "bolus," and he was unaware that he was speaking to a relatively inexperienced nurse; the new nurse did not recall and did not check for drug administration, dosage, routes and time, and dilution required for KCl, and operated from a stance of ignorance or lack of memory about KCl and blindly adhering to a physician's order without verifying its reasonableness and safety before administering the drug.

Nurse Murphy is responsible for knowing that a concentrated intravenous dose of KCl is lethal and is equally responsible for looking up an unfamiliar drug before administering it. She did not perceive her professional responsibility to verify the accuracy and safety of all medical orders before carrying out the order. This error occurred before KCl was assigned "red alert" status and made unavailable in concentrated doses on nursing units. These "system" corrections would have closed a crucial hole in the system "Swiss cheese" alignment and prevented this tragic error. Professional responsibility and accountability require that Nurse Murphy look up the indications, dangers, and actions of KCl as required by the Model Administrative Rules (NCSBN, 2004). Nurse Murphy maintains her nursing license and has not incurred further practice problems, her evaluations have been positive in a new place of employment, and she states that she carries a drug reference book with her at all times.

CONCLUSIONS

These case histories raise persistent questions as to the reasons the nurses were not quick to communicate with primary care physicians and referring physicians. To what extent do communication barriers exist, and is this barrier interpersonal, interprofessional, or physical in nature? Why didn't the nurse check drug references for information about KCl before administering it? Is pharmacologic information readily available to nursing staff, and if so, is it sought and used? What remedial and regulatory actions are appropriate when a nurse is not cognizant of her lack of knowledge? Institutional in-service education should be stressing the importance of routing verification and checking of the safety of all health care provider orders, and this should be an absolute requirement verified by a reporting system for *new* health care provider orders. A lack of institutional responsibility for patient safety is demonstrated by the lack of these ongoing patient safety education measures. These two cases affirm an educational gap in preparing nurses to safely make a case for a physician order and following through with verification, and then checking the safety and appropriateness of the physician order. Active ongoing inquiry of all professionals is paramount to patient safety (see Cullen et al., 1997).

The safe administration of medications and ongoing investigation of medication errors to design the system to better support accurate medication administration, and ongoing continuing education of all health care professionals on the administration of medications, are all required to improve patient safety in the administration of medications. As Henriksen et al. (2008) point out, human factors research is needed in all areas of nursing practice but especially in the area of the administration of medications:

Many nursing work processes have evolved as a result of local practice or personal preference rather than through a systematic approach of designing a system that leads to fewer errors and greater efficiency. Far too often, providers and administrators have fallen into a "status quo trap," doing things simply because they always have been done that way. Human factors practitioners, on the other hand, take into account human strengths and weaknesses in the design of systems, emphasizing the importance of avoiding reliance on memory, vigilance, and follow-up intentions—areas where human performance is less reliable. Key processes can be simplified and standardized, which leads to less confusion, gains in efficiency, and fewer errors. When care processes become standardized, nurses have more time to attend to individual patients' specialized needs, which typically are not subject to standardization. When medical devices and new technology are designed with the end user in mind, ease of use and error detection or preventability are possible, in contrast to many current "opaque" computer-controlled devices that prevent the provider from understanding their full functionality (Henriksen et al., 2008, p. 2).

Evaluating practice breakdown and system redesign and specifically designed educational efforts will reduce medication errors. Ongoing quality improvement is a professional responsibility that requires ongoing examination and reexamination of the contributions made by the system, health care community member, and nurse in regarding each practice breakdown event that occurs (Wolf, 1994). Individual, practice communities, and systems of health care delivery must all receive adequate ongoing quality improvement efforts to improve patient safety.

References

Agency for Healthcare Research and Quality. (2008). Medical errors and patient safety. Available online at http://www.ahrq.gov/qual/errorsix.htm. Retrieved October 1, 2008.

Benner, P., Sutphen, M., Leonard-Kahn, V., Day, L. (In press.) *Educating nurses: A call for radical transformation.* San Francisco: Jossey-Bass and Carnegie Foundation for the Advancement of Teaching.

Cullen, D. J., Sweitzer, B. J., Bates, D. W., Burdick, E., Edmondson, A., & Leape, L. L. (1997). Preventable adverse drug events in hospitalized patients: A comparative study of intensive care and general care units. *Critical Care Medicine, 25*(8), 1289-1297.

Ely, J., Levinson, W., Elder, N., Mainous, A., Vinson, D. (1995). Perceived causes of family physicians' errors. *Journal of Family Practice, 40*(4), 337-344.

Gladstone, J. (1995). Drug administration errors: a study into the factors underlying the occurrence and reporting of drug errors in a district general hospital. *Journal of Advanced Nursing, 22*(4), 628-637.

Henriksen, K., Dayton, E., Keyes, M. A., Caravon, P., & Hughes, R. (2008). Understanding adverse events: a human factors framework. In R. Hughes (Ed.), *Patient safety and quality: A handbook for nurses* (pp. 1-19). Rockville, MD: Agency for Healthcare Policy and Research.

Hughes, R. (Ed.). (2008). *Patient safety and quality: A handbook for nurses.* Rockville, MD: Agency for Healthcare Policy and Research. Available online at http://www.ahrq.gov/qual/nurseshndbk/. Retrieved 8/15/08.

Institute of Safe Medication Practices (ISMP). (2008). Available online at http://www.ismp.org/Pages/ismp_erract.html. Retrieved October 30, 2008.

The Joint Commission. (2008). Available online at www.JointCommission.org. Retrieved October 30, 2008.

Kohn, L. T., Corrigan, J. M., & Donaldson, M. S (Eds.); Committee on Quality of Health Care in America, Institute of Medicine. (2000). *To err is human: Building a safer health system.* Washington, DC: The National Academies Press.

Maddox, P. J., Wakefield, M., & Bull, J. (2001). Patient safety and the need for professional and educational change. *Nursing Outlook, 49*(1), 8-13.

National Council of State Boards of Nursing (NCSBN). (2004). Model nursing administrative rules. The NCSVN Model Nursing Practice Act and Model Nursing Administrative Rules were revised by the 2004 Delegate Assembly. See http://www.ncsbn.org/1455.htm.

Ohioans First. (2004; 2009). Available online at http://www.ohiopatientsafety.org/meds/. Retrieved June 15, 2009.

Page, A (Ed.); Committee on the Work Environment for Nurses and Patient Safety, Institute of Medicine. (2004). *Keeping patients safe: Transforming the work environment for nurses.* Washington, D.C.: The National Academies Press.

Reason, J. (1990). *Human error.* Cambridge: Cambridge University Press.

Weick, K. E., & Sutcliffe, K. M. (2001). *Managing the unexpected: Assuring high performance in an age of complexity.* San Francisco: Jossey-Bass.

Williams, C. (2004). Inside a closed-loop medication strategy. *Nursing Management, 35* (Suppl. 5), 8-9, 24.

Wolf, Z. R. (1994). *Medication errors: The nursing experience.* Albany, NY: Delmar.

3

Practice Breakdown: Clearly Communicating Patient Data and Clinical Assessments

Kathy Malloch ◆ *Linda Patterson* ◆ *Vickie Sheets* ◆ *Karen Bowen*

Chapter Outline

ISSUES IN NURSING DOCUMENTATION

Health care requires good teamwork. Nursing care can never occur in isolation. Communication is central. Written documentation and clear presentations of "making a case" for patient intervention are core competencies of nurses. Perhaps nowhere is system design more important than in documentation. A system must be designed with the goals of the practice of all health care team members, the patient's well-being and safety, and in the context of the actual work environment. A good system of documentation can improve practice, while a poor one may hinder practice.

The purpose of documentation is to clearly communicate the condition of the patient as well as the assessment, planning, implementation, and evaluation work of nursing. It is a continual and ongoing process that reflects the changing needs and conditions of the patient. Documentation is the critical and sometimes only form of communication among all health care providers about the current condition of a patient.

Currently patient care documentation is found in a variety of forms and formats, handwritten and computerized. Written documentation systems have been developed to assist clinicians to produce accurate and comprehensive documentation. Examples include the following: (a) problem-intervention-evaluation charting (PIE); (b) subjective-objective-assessment-plan charting

(SOAP); (c) problem-oriented medical record charting (POMR); and (d) charting by exception formats, outcome-based charting; and critical pathways (Meiner, 1999). Checklists for exception charting to address the time restraints have been implemented as documentation requirements for regulatory compliance increase. At times, nurses shortcut documentation because of time constraints or limitations of these forms at the expense of complete charting.

As patient care becomes increasingly complex, the importance of timely and accurate documentation becomes increasingly important. Delays, omissions, and errors in documentation may result in delays or errors in assessments, interventions, treatments, procedures, and medication administration. These errors often create a cascade of events that may negatively impact patient care or patient outcome.

DOCUMENTATION OF THE FUTURE

The written documentation record will increasingly appear in the form of an electronic record. The structure, organization, and retrieval of patient data must be user friendly and secure, and should be designed with the workflow of those documenting their patient care in mind. Computerized documentation systems are more than automation of existing paper forms. State-of-the-art documentation systems are designed to more closely reflect the flow of patient care processes in an orderly way and to increase patient safety within the available features and design. Computerized clinical documentation systems that support functional requirements contribute significantly to patient safety and caregiver effectiveness.

Significant advantages for safe patient care can be realized as electronic systems are implemented across the country. Safe nursing practice is supported in the following ways with an electronic record that includes:

1. Design of documentation systems that more closely reflect actual work processes and patient throughput, supporting clinician assessments and work organization
2. Integration of physician order entry, medication administration, and clinician documentation systems
3. Inclusion of a framework that encompasses nursing knowledge functions as a cognitive map for clinicians (nurses handle large amounts of data and often experience overload and stress; also provides professional support in making complex clinical decisions) and increases efficiency (von Krogh et al., 2005)
4. Integration of standards-based organizing frameworks such as Nursing Interventions (NIC), Nursing Outcomes (NOC), and North American Nursing Diagnosis Association (NANDA)
5. Use of a complex and comprehensive database for patient and nursing research

6. Inclusion of alerts, popups, and protocols to guide caregivers in both care processes and documentation

Specific outcomes from computerized documentation that have an impact on patient safety and decrease the potential for practice breakdown include:

1. Elimination of illegibility
2. Minimized duplication
3. Improved response time to patient requests
4. Simultaneous, real-time access to up-to-date patient data for multiple clinicians
5. Improved documentation completeness
6. Increased compliance with regulatory requirements (e.g., assessments for pain level, skin integrity, and fall risk)

Users often develop "shortcuts" and "work-arounds" for a poorly designed system of documentation that does not take into account the workflow processes or the time required for documenting. For example, if there are rigid rules for documenting the administration of medications within one-half hour of administration, and the patient-to-nurse ratio is too high, the nurse may be tempted to document before actually administering the medication. This sets the patient up for undetected "missed doses" of medication. Also, if the workflow and patient care record are poorly designed, requiring excessive amounts of time for access, then nurses may not have a chance to document their assessments and treatments in a timely manner. Nondocumented therapies place patients at great risk for second doses of narcotics, sedatives, or other medications.

The importance of documentation becomes apparent following reviews of incidents in which a patient has been affected negatively. Not surprisingly, documentation is rarely the primary error. The down side of the extensive requirements for documentation in today's complex hospitals is that the nurse can spend from 13% to 28% of his or her time in patient care documentation, and this reduction in the nurses' availability to provide direct patient care has been shown to diminish patient safety (Korst et al., 2003; Pabst et al., 1996; Page, 2004).

KEY PRINCIPLES

Key principles regarding documentation indicate that documentation of the current status of the patient is needed and includes assessment, care plan updates, implementation, and evaluation of care provided, and that documentation is a critical task that nurses perform to protect the patient.

The following is a case study in which documentation played a role in the practice breakdown of nursing care. The story is encapsulated for the reader with a sample of the actual documentation provided by the nurses involved. The reader is encouraged to question whether the documentation truly reflects the story presented.

HISTORICAL CASE STUDY #1: Late and Later Documentation

PRACTICE BREAKDOWN IN DOCUMENTATION

Ms. Amy Jones was a 55-year-old woman being treated for depression at a mental health facility. She was alert, oriented, ambulating without difficulty, and interacting appropriately with staff. The patient's family was scheduled for a meeting with her treatment team in the afternoon. During the day Ms. Jones met with her psychiatrist, Dr. Ian Smith, in Ms. Jones's room. When her roommate came in, Dr. Smith suggested that they complete their session in his office, and Ms. Jones accompanied him to that space. On the way she complained that she felt weak but could make it. During the session she reported that she had a headache, which Dr. Smith attributed to anxiety. He went to look for a nurse to provide medication for Ms. Jones. On his return with Ms. Mary Sullivan, a registered nurse, Ms. Jones was on the floor on her knees vomiting. A physician working across the hall came and assisted Dr. Smith and Nurse Sullivan with Ms. Jones, who was now quite somnolent, into a wheelchair. Dr. Allen, the primary care physician, ordered that Ms. Jones be given Phenergan IM for the vomiting and that the nursing staff monitor her bowel sounds. Dr. Allen reported that she was not informed of Ms. Jones' complaints of headache or loss of bowel control. Dr. Allen thought that she was dealing with gastrointestinal symptoms so she had the nurses check for bowel sounds and softness of the patient's belly. She reports that she received a second callback and was told bowel sounds were normal, the patient's stomach was soft, and the patient was resting comfortably. Ms. Jones was bathed and returned to her bed. She took the prescribed Phenergan after which she vomited several more times during that shift. She was incontinent of stool once. No one considered conducting neurologic checks because the staff thought Ms. Jones was suffering from a virus.

When Ms. Jones's family members arrived, the nurses advised them that their mother was sick and was sleeping, and would not be able to attend the meeting. The family members could not arouse the patient. The staff said that Ms. Jones had been administered Phenergan for vomiting and would be awake by evening. Family members returned that evening and found the patient still unresponsive with vomit in her mouth. The family checked Ms. Jones' pupils and found them unequal. The family reported to the registered nurse at the desk, and another nurse checked Ms. Jones' vital signs and reported them to be normal. The family telephoned Ms. Jones' primary care physician, Dr. Allen, and the nurse gave him a report. Soon after this call, an ambulance transported Ms. Jones to the hospital for evaluation. Ms. Jones subsequently died at the hospital.

Ms. Jones' daughter stated that the registered nurse did not assess her mother; on arrival in the unit, the EMT assessed Ms. Jones. Ms. Jones' daughter did not believe that her mother had been adequately monitored from noon to 6:30 PM.

She also complained that the nurses were laughing at the family's concerns about the condition in which they found their mother.

Ms. Cherie Hoffman, a registered nurse, had been employed at the facility for 25 years. She began her career as a nursing assistant, a title she held for 7 years. She then served as a licensed practical nurse for 10 years and then as a registered nurse for the past 6 years. She was familiar with all of the policies and procedures of the facility. On the day of the event Ms. Hoffman was working as the charge nurse; she noted that it was a particularly busy day. She returned from lunch and was informed by Nurse Sullivan that Ms. Jones was ill and had vomited. She was bathed, and the staff had documented her vital signs, completed the Glucoscan, and medicated Ms. Jones with Phenergan per Dr. Allen's order. The family was not notified of a change in Ms. Jones' condition because they were expected for a family conference at 3 PM, and Nurse Sullivan hoped that Ms. Jones would feel better by then and could participate in the conference. Nurse Hoffman assisted Nurse Sullivan in monitoring Ms. Jones throughout the rest of the shift. Nurse Hoffman had understood that Ms. Jones had not been sleeping well and thought it would be good to let her sleep. Nurse Hoffman thought Nurse Sullivan had last assessed Ms. Jones at 7 PM.

Nurse Hoffman states she was never informed that Ms. Jones had collapsed prior to vomiting or that she had a headache, or that Ms. Jones was somnolent after the episode. She reported that Ms. Jones had a history of headaches, nausea, and dizziness, all of which had been attributed to medications.

Nurse Sullivan recalls reporting everything to Nurse Hoffman. Nurse Sullivan said she had checked bowel sounds as directed. Ms. Jones was incontinent of stool at 2 PM. and was bathed and repositioned. Around 6 PM. Nurse Sullivan straightened Ms. Jones in bed and said that Ms. Jones looked comfortable. Nurse Sullivan said that she did not feel anxious about the patient, as she thought Ms. Jones was sleeping. Ms. Jones was not on 15-minute checks, but Nurse Sullivan recalled checking on Ms. Jones frequently throughout the shift to assess for vomiting.

Dr. Smith stated that, in retrospect, he should have personally talked to Dr. Allen about Ms. Jones's condition and communicated to Nurse Sullivan that Ms. Jones had complained about a headache prior to the episode.

PATIENT MEDICAL RECORD: PROGRESS NOTES (ORIGINAL ENTRY AT 7 PM)

O/B client showered and met with Dr. While out with physician, client had episode of vomiting small amounts. Over a period of 30 minutes, client was medicated with Phenergan. Client was later incontinent of a moderate amount of stool. Assisted with activities of daily living (ADLs). Notified Dr. of situation. No further change in Dr.'s orders. Continues to be unresponsive. Physically ill today. Keep MD informed of changes.

Registered Nurse Sullivan

ADDENDUM TO PROGRESS NOTES, DATED TWO DAYS LATER (MEDICAL RECORD ENTRY)

Received a call to assists client in Dr.'s office; client lying on floor, diaphoretic, reported to have felt weak, nauseated, dizzy. Client started to vomit. Assisted and supported client while she vomited 3 times. Two assisted to wheelchair then back to bed—minimal efforts given by patient with transfer. VS, 12:20 97.2 64 16 134/72 (patient lying down). Reported to charge nurse, client changed and washed. Lung sounds assessed, clear all lobes. Phenergan given at 12:20, blood sugar check at 12:30. Rails up, client on right side. 13:00 noticed to have vomited again. Charge nurse notified, vomitus clear yellow with odor. Charge nurse assisted with cleaning patient. Bowel sounds assessed, low gurgling in 4 abdominal quadrants, info given to charge nurse. 14:00 checks. Client noted to be incontinent of stools. Bathed and repositioned. Pulse 60 reg. & even, respirations unlabored, blood sugar done at 16:20. Client repositioned. During checks from 1800-1900 patient's head had moved, repositioned. Pulse rechecked 56 reg. & even, all clothing washed and hung to dry. A medical change with nausea and tiredness. Charge nurse and MD notified of all information.

Registered Nurse Sullivan

NURSING NOTES (ADDENDUM TO ORIGINAL ENTRY THREE DAYS LATER) (MEDICAL RECORD ENTRY)

I returned from lunch. Another nurse on staff reported to me that Ms. Jones had an episode of vomiting and had to be assisted to bed, to be medicated. After about 15 min, I went into patient's room. She appeared to be sleeping. I called Dr.'s office and gave the information to some person. Later Dr. returned call and I explained that the patient had vomited several times. I also told Dr. that the patient appeared unresponsive but also informed her that she had been medicated. I gave her a complete set of vital signs and blood sugar. Dr. expressed concern re a possible abdominal problem and asked me to be sure I checked for bowel sounds. I called Dr. a second time to report the situation and told her that bowel sounds were present and that the patient had defecated. Stool was soft, formed, no further vomiting, and the patient continued to be unresponsive; breathing appeared normal (later call received from Dr.'s office regarding condition). I repeated the previous information. Patient was checked q 15 min all day with staff checking and carefully paying attention to be sure that the patient had not vomited any further. She was turned and appeared comfortable. When the patient's daughter came in to visit, I informed her of her mother's vomiting and explained that she had been medicated and was sleeping at that time approx 1500. Family returned at approx 1900 and became quite upset and insisted a Dr. be called. The physician on call at that time ordered the patient to be transferred to ER for medical evaluation. This was done at 1930.

Registered Nurse Hoffman

FACILITY ACTION

Nurse Hoffman was placed on 3-month performance probation. This probation was extended for further observation of assessment skills. Subsequently it was determined that competency in this area was still a problem, and her employment was terminated. Nurse Sullivan was allowed to resign in lieu of termination (termination would have been a result of ongoing performance problems related to nursing assessment and documentation).

NURSING BOARD/COMMISSION ACTION

Registered Nurse Hoffman and Registered Nurse Sullivan voluntarily allowed permanent revocation of their registered nurse licenses without admission of violation and without admission to any alleged facts.

ANALYSIS OF CASE STUDY #1

1. This case departs from nursing standards specifically as there were (a) failures to accurately assess and document the patient's condition and (b) failures to notify/accurately report change in the patient's condition to the physician. In particular, the patient's decreased level of alertness was not accurately conveyed with relevant questions and interpretations.

   a. *An acceptable level of performance.* The nurse instituted physician orders and monitored the patient during her change in condition. The nurse documented the medications administered, patient vomiting, and bowel status.

   b. *An unacceptable level of performance.* The level of medical review and examination was inadequate on the part of the psychiatrist, Dr. Smith, and the patient's primary care physician, Dr. Allen. Neither doctor performed even a minimum level of physical examination, evaluation of neurologic status, or followed through on the patient's "overreaction" to Phenergan.

   c. *An unacceptable level of performance.* The nurses' ongoing assessment and communication of the patient's deteriorating condition was inadequate. The nurses were not adequately attentive to the puzzling situation of the patient remaining somnolent for so long, nor did the nurses conduct a neurologic check on the patient. The nurses did not obtain complete information from the physician regarding precipitating events prior to the acute illness episode. Poor communication between the physician and the nurses and failure to document and communicate these concerns to the primary physician resulted in a misdiagnosis and inappropriate treatment of the patient. Specifically, the failure was that the staff did not completely document and communicate the patient's condition, which included (1) incontinence, (2) decreased level of consciousness, (3) no neurologic checks, (4) finding the patient on the floor, and (5) diaphoretic state. There was a failure to document the ongoing assessments, and the monitoring and evaluation of interventions implemented. Finally, late entries of documentations of significant interventions and assessments meant that these assessments were not available to other members of the team during the incident.

2. System issues focused on (a) leadership, (b) workforce, (c) work processes, and (d) organizational culture.

    a. Leadership

       1) Lack of process regarding communication between psychiatrist and primary care physician resulting in poor coordination of care.

       2) Lack of policy on complete assessments and documentation of patients following a change in patient's physical and mental condition.

    b. Experienced workforce. Leadership was not adequately monitoring workforce skills and competency. A review of the incident and monitoring actions found that knowledge and performance deficits were noted for both nurses resulting in their termination and resignation.

    c. Work processes. The investigation found that a process was not in place to ensure coverage during lunch, and there was a breakdown in formal communication among staff. No one nurse was identified as "assigned" to assume total responsibility for the patient.

    d. Organizational culture. The investigation results indicated a lack of clear, concise communication and a multidisciplinary approach with poor coordination of care.

3. *Individual Nurse Issues.* Nurse Hoffman was responsible for the entire unit. She received a report on a change in the patient's condition. She did not get a full and complete report from Nurse Sullivan and failed to collaborate with the physician. She called the primary physician and relayed the incomplete information to the physician. It would have been preferable for Nurse Sullivan to call the physician because she had made a direct assessment of the patient and was best able to communicate the patient's condition and answer any questions. Nurse Hoffman stated that she monitored the patient during the shift. She failed to document the monitoring or describe what her monitoring entailed.

4. *Practice Responsibilities.* The practice responsibilities expected in this situation included (a) an assessment of the patient, (b) documentation of the assessment, (c) a plan to address the patient's needs that included coordination with the multidisciplinary team, (d) steps to implement the physician's orders and measures to ensure ongoing nursing assessments of the patient's responses to the medication given, (e) an evaluation of the patient's response to care, documented along with a report of any changes or deviations from expected outcomes; and (f) measures to initiate the process over again. In this situation, the patient needed to be sent to the emergency room earlier for physical assessment or examined initially by the primary care physician, preferably in the psychiatrist's office, and at the time the patient returned to the unit incapacitated.

Clearly the entire staff was not thinking about the possibilities that the patient could have a serious condition other than her psychological condition and the hypothesized "virus," abdominal problems, or high blood sugar levels. Psychiatric facilities have a "set" to think about psychiatric problems rather than medical-surgical problems. Both physicians and the nurses failed to conduct adequate assessments given the level of Ms. Jones signs and symptoms. Curiosity and vigilance were lacking with regard to Ms. Jones puzzling deterioration, and adequate documentation of signs and symptoms and the continued somnolence and deterioration of the patient were not adequately reported or documented. This tragic case is a signal event that must be highlighted in the psychiatric facility in order to improve nursing and physician assessments of patients for medical conditions and to avoid a repeated dangerous selective focus on psychiatric problems only.

ADDITIONAL EXAMPLES

Following are other examples of documentation that do not conform to nursing standards of documentation:

Nurse Daniels reported to work for her evening shift. She was told by the day shift that there was an admission expected that evening. She was informed that one of the other nurses had called in sick. She considered calling the house supervisor and requesting more staff but decided against it. She assessed the situation and tried to prioritize her responsibilities for the shift.

Nurse Daniels told herself that if she hurried and cut a few corners she would be able to handle the workload. She started her evening administration of medications. She decided it would save time if she signed all of the Medication Administration Records (MARs) first, then administered the medications to patients. She was familiar with all of the patients and the medications they received in the evening so this made sense to her. She went through the MARs and signed all of the evening medications. She was about halfway through administering medications to patients when she became nauseated and diaphoretic. She started vomiting. Another nurse took her temperature and called her husband to come and drive her home.

The house supervisor was informed of the situation and assigned Nurse Martin, a float nurse, to cover for Nurse Daniels. Nurse Martin reviewed the MARs and determined the evening medications had all been passed out before Nurse Daniels became ill and had to leave. Later in the shift, some of the patients reported they had not received their evening medications. Nurse Martin was in an impossible situation of trying to determine who had and who had not received their medications.

Although well intended, Nurse Daniels' actions resulted in several medication omissions including blood pressure medications, antibiotics, and blood thinners.

What seemed to be a harmless shortcut turned out to be dangerous. Hospitals are complex environments with many interruptions. Documentation is a major line of defense for patient safety. Omitting documentation or documenting prior to actual interventions puts patients in jeopardy.

In another situation, Nurse Cross was assigned to perform blood sugar Accu-Check monitoring for the shift on her unit. After she completed all of the Accu-Check monitoring, she referred to her notes and charted the values in her patients' records. She realized she must have written the results for the patient, Ms. Nancy Bruno, on a separate piece of paper that was not in her uniform pocket but was rather on another note that she had left in the medication room. She felt fairly certain that she remembered it to be 280. This violates a patient safety precaution against relying on memory for laboratory values, dosages, or even normal ranges, etc. The nurse was in a hurry and recorded the 280, intending to find her other note and double-check the number. Meanwhile she became busy and forgot to check for the actual correct number. Ms. Bruno was a patient on a sliding scale for her insulin. Nurse Brown was passing out medications during that shift. She noted the 280 and administered insulin accordingly. Ms. Bruno's Accu-Check was actually 180, and consequently too much insulin was given for the blood sugar level. Ms. Bruno had a reaction and required administration of glucagon and close monitoring.

Again, although Nurse Cross had good intentions, she cut corners and did not follow nursing standards for medication administration. As a result, Ms. Bruno was put at serious risk and suffered an unnecessary adverse reaction.

SUMMARY

Documentation is a contested area of nursing practice. Nurses complain that they spend too much time on documentation and that their work demands often preclude timely charting. Keenan et al. (2008) identified the following key research questions for documentation:

1. How does variability in documentation impact patient outcomes?
2. What are the key components of an effective documentation process that is patient centered and improves the transfer of information among clinicians and across settings of care?
3. What aspects of documentation are shared among an interdisciplinary team, and what contributions to the patient record can each team member effectively provide?
4. Should documentation vary across settings of care (Keenan et al., 2008)?

The TERCAP® tool can add address post hoc patterns of documentation that are associated with poor patient outcomes. False documentation to cover up any kind of error is a serious breach of nursing professional standards and is reportable to the state board of nursing. Likewise "late charting," especially several days after the event, is highly problematic and prone to error, and hindsight filling in information that was not discerned or known at the time of the unfolding of an event is a serious breach of professional standards. Keenan et al. (2008) concluded that we have a long way to go in improving the design and safety and quality improvement of nursing documentation and planning of patient care. After their extensive literature review, they drew the following conclusions:

> The evidence reviewed in this chapter suggests that formal recordkeeping practices (documentation into the medical record) are failing to fulfill their primary purpose, of supporting information flow that ensures the continuity, quality, and safety of care. Moreover, disproportionate attention to secondary purposes (e.g., accreditation and legal standards) has produced a medical record that is document centered rather than patient focused. Cumbersome and variable formats, useless content, poor accessibility, and shadow records are all evidence of the extraordinary failure of the medical record. Given the exorbitant cost of the record and urgent need for tools that facilitate the flow of patient-centric information within and across systems, it is imperative to develop broad-based solutions.

The TERCAP database from the state board of nursing will potentially provide a useful source of data on the impact of nursing documentation on serious reportable nursing errors that come to the state board of nursing.

References

Keenan, G. M., Yakel, E., Tschannen, D., & Mandeville, M. (2008). Documentation and the nurse care planning process. In R. Hughes (Ed.), *Patient safety and quality: A handbook for nurses* (pp. 1-33). Rockville, MD: Agency for Healthcare Policy and Research. Available online at www.ahrq.gov/qual/nurseshdbk/. Accessed 10-30-2008.

Korst, L., Eusebio-Angeja, A., Chamorrow, T., Aydin, C., & Gregory, K. (2003). Nursing documentation time during implementation of an electronic medical record. *Journal of the American Medical Association, 33*(1), 24-30.

Meiner, S. (1999). *Nursing documentation: Legal focus across practice settings.* Thousand Oaks, CA: Sage.

Pabst, M., Scherubel, J., & Minnick, A. (1996). The impact of computerized documentation on nurses' use of time. *Computers in Nursing, 14*(1), 25-30.

Page, A. (Ed.); Committee on the Work Environment for Nurses and Patient Safety, Institute of Medicine. (2004). *Keeping patients safe: Transforming the work environment of nurses.* Washington, DC: The National Academies Press.

von Krogh, G., Dale, C., & Naden, D. (2005). A framework for integrating NANDA, NIC, and NOC terminology in electronic patient records. *Journal of Nursing Scholarship, 37*(3), 275-281.

4

Practice Breakdown: Attentiveness/Surveillance

Karla Bitz ♦ *Vicki Goettsche* ♦ *Patricia Benner*

Chapter Outline

The nursing shortage has created multiple changes within the nursing profession leading to diminished nurse-patient contact and less attention to the needs of patients. Fewer nursing caregivers are available today to provide nursing care to a more acutely ill patient population and lower nurse-to-patient staffing ratios have been shown to decrease patient safety (Aiken et al., 2003; Cho et al., 2003).

The goal of system designers is to minimize the attentiveness required of human beings with the caveats that even the best-designed systems require intelligent human alertness and attentiveness to deviations in the performance and design flaws of these systems. In complex, open-ended, underdetermined systems such as health care, attentiveness and critical thinking cannot be engineered out of the system (Weick and Sutcliff, 2001). In fact, the loss of transparency that accompanies increased automation and technology calls for even more attentive monitoring and thoughtfulness on the part of professionals (Reason, 1990).

Health care systems must be designed to foster attentiveness to the most important critical aspects in the clinical situation while "disenburdening" the human problem solvers and knowledge workers. As noted by the Institute of

Medicine (IOM) report "Keeping Patients Safe: Transforming the Work Environment of Nurses" (Page, 2004):

> A primary activity performed by nursing staff in all hospitals, long-term care facilities, and ambulatory settings is ongoing patient surveillance (sometimes referred to as patient "assessment," "evaluation," or "monitoring")—an important mechanism for the detection of errors and the prevention of adverse events. If a patient's status begins to decline, the decline will be detectable though the nurse's observation of changes in the patient's physical or cognitive status. Performance of this patient monitoring requires great attention, knowledge, and responsiveness on the part of the nurse (Page, 2004, p. 32).

A major threat to attentiveness and surveillance for all health care workers is sleep deprivation and fatigue. Shift work is required in hospitals, long-term care, rehabilitation, and psychiatric facilities—that is, in any institution where around-the-clock care is required. Coffey, Skipper, and Jung (1988) report that hospitals usually have 8-hour and 12-hour shifts, with slightly more than one third of all nurses working on shifts other than day shifts. This report was completed in 1988, and since that time patient acuity in hospitals has required increased staffing on evening and night shifts. With staff shortages, the problem of fatigue and sleep deprivation can become compounded by nurses working extra shifts. Four disasters, the Exxon Valdez, Bhopal, Chernobyl, and Three Mile Island have been associated with sleep deprivation and fatigue, as have driving and airline accidents (Mitler et al., 1988; Rosekind et al., 2004; Wylie et al., 1996). The quality of sleep deteriorates with disturbed sleep-wake patterns, and chronic disturbances in sleep cycles often cause cumulative sleep deprivation (Smith-Coggins et al., 1994; 1997; 2006; Smith-Coggins & Rosekind, 2004). Quiet shifts on long-term care units may create negative patterns of "dozing" and inattentiveness due to fatigue.

Vigilance on the part of nurses is required in order to anticipate and respond to predictable complications, to monitor changes in the patient's condition, and to handle unpredictable emergency conditions that may arise. A commercial and competitive environment in health care increases emphasis on efficiency without equal emphasis on effectiveness, which further increases the demands for nurses' focus and attention while creating climates that make attentiveness to particular patient needs more difficult. Efficiency, if it disrupts attentiveness, is not efficient because it is ineffective. Performing more and more interventions at a faster pace impedes life-saving attentiveness.

To cope with the high demands of work overload, nurses use risky shortcuts because they have too many competing demands for their attention and lack the system supports that they need to provide safe, reliable care. Efficiency, shortcuts, and productivity may be the major organizational source of rewards and recognition while the consequences of inattentiveness may go unrecognized. Attentiveness and surveillance to the patient's well-being and changing condition provide an essential first-line defense against undetected changes in the patient's condition and hazards in the administration of therapies as well as environmental hazards in the hospital. The good outcomes of adequate levels of nurse attentiveness typically go unmeasured, and we are left with indirect measures of the absence of adequate attentiveness to the patient's needs. It is easy to identify a problem with inattentiveness when the patient goes unchecked or unmonitored for long periods of time. It is more difficult to identify problems with rushed assessments and interventions.

Nurses who observe their colleagues cutting corners in ways that might endanger patient safety are expected to speak directly to the nurse or report their concerns to management or administration (Maxfield et al., 2005). However, when staff perceives that punitive or even nonconstructive communication will result, there will be less incentive to report such incidents since punitive reprimands rather than constructive problem-solving may only make the problem worse. Mustard (2002) describes a culture of patient safety that focuses on improving system issues. Poor system design and short staffing interfere with attentiveness. A culture of safety is achieved by building one that encourages mutual disclosure and immediate corrective action without the anxiety of blame and shame. A sense of collective responsibility and continuing improvement and a just social climate are central to improving the quality and effectiveness of nursing attentiveness to patients' changing conditions and needs.

Recommendation 6-2 of the IOM report (Page, 2004) discusses the direct-care nursing efforts and the nursing leadership that are necessary in order to reduce errors. Those direct-care efforts include attentiveness and observant surveillance of a patient's health status. Lack of recognition or detection of patient care needs jeopardizes all patients but is especially dangerous for patients who are very young, heavily medicated, somnolent, unconscious, or cognitively impaired. Table 4.1 describes the practice breakdown category of attentiveness and surveillance. If the nurse has not observed the patient, then he/she cannot determine whether changes have occurred and/or make knowledgeable decisions about the patient.

STAFFING ISSUES AND ATTENTIVENESS

The nursing shortage has had a significant impact on nurses' ability to provide safe patient care. Working short-staffed or understaffed, requiring mandatory overtime, and working long hours and possibly two jobs are just a few of the

TABLE **4.1 Case Analysis Category of Breakdown: Attentiveness/TERCAP® Surveillance Items**

Cause of Breakdown	Examples
Absence of patient contact or monitoring	Patient not observed for an unsafe period of time
	Staff performance not observed for an unsafe period of time

results of the nursing shortage. Numerous studies and summaries of the impact of nurse staffing on patient outcomes have documented the seriousness and far-reaching nature of problems associated with the nursing shortage. In a recent study conducted by Needleman et al. (2002) about nurse staffing levels and quality of care issues in hospitals, they reported that a higher proportion of hours of nursing care provided by registered nurses and a greater number of hours of care by registered nurses per day were directly associated with better care for hospitalized patients.

Aiken et al. (2002) found that nurses in hospitals with the highest patient-to-nurse ratios are more than twice as likely to experience job-related burnout and almost twice as likely to be dissatisfied with their jobs compared to nurses in the hospitals with the lowest patient-to-nurse ratios. Aiken and colleagues also noted that inadequate staffing is one of the factors that adversely affects the quality of health care and negatively impacts patient care and safety (Aiken et al., 2003). The relationship of nurse staffing levels with the rescue of patients with life-threatening conditions suggests that nurses contribute significantly to surveillance, early detection, and timely interventions that save lives (Aiken et al., 2002).

Inadequate staffing also fosters practice breakdown and compromises the safety of the patients, nurses, and other staff. Nurses who are working short-staffed may not have the time to perform their responsibilities in a careful manner and may not be able to identify the subtle but life-threatening changes in a patient's condition. Nurses are present around the clock to detect complications in patients and initiate prompt interventions to minimize negative outcomes (Clarke & Aiken, 2003). Aiken et al. (2003) determined that patients in hospitals with a higher proportion of nurses educated at the baccalaureate level or higher had patients that actually experienced lower mortality and failure-to-rescue rates than hospitals with fewer baccalaureate and advanced-practice nurses. In this particular study, *failure to rescue* was defined as "death within thirty days among patients who experienced complications" (Aiken et al., 2003, p. 4).

SYSTEMS AND ATTENTIVENESS

In addition to the availability of nurses, the organizational structures and issues related to system processes within the health care environment also affect the attentiveness or inattentiveness of nurses. For example, environmental issues of increased noise levels, poor lighting, or equipment failures within the work setting can impede attentiveness and alter the competencies of interventions by nurses (Ulrich et al., 2004).

> When people are hospitalized, in a nursing home, having a baby, or learning to manage a chronic condition in their own homes—at some of their most vulnerable moments—nurses are the health care providers they are most likely to encounter; spend the greatest amount of time with and . . . depend on for their recovery" (Page, 2004, p. 2).

Hospitalized patients require close monitoring and rapid adjustment of therapies. Acutely ill patients are physiologically unstable and require patient, response-based interventions and monitoring for untoward effects of both the ongoing therapies and disease states.

Nurses, the primary caregivers, are present with patients more than any other health care professional. Patients place their trust for the safety of their lives in a nurse's hands when they are the sickest and the most vulnerable. Nurses are expected to be attentive to patients' changing conditions and to act in the best interests of their patients. Patient safety depends on nurses paying attention to patients' clinical conditions and responses to therapies, as well as potential hazards or errors in treatment (Benner et al., 2002).

TECHNOLOGY AND ATTENTIVENESS

The significance of the nurse's role in monitoring technical interventions has also increased as modern medicine has increased the level of technology. Patient safety requires that nurses understand and monitor for complications such as proliferating new surgeries, interventional radiology, electrophysiologic interventions, and highly technical care for premature infants. Nurses take on an increasingly vital role in detecting and ensuring early intervention in the progression of their patients' illnesses and responses to treatment.

The numbers of technical health care interventions per patient have increased in hospitals, in skilled nursing facilities, and in the home. Patients receive an array of pharmaceutical products with potential for drug interactions. Many pharmaceutical interventions must be titrated according to the patient's physiologic responses to the drug(s). Nurses monitor patients' responses to the intravenous therapies whose therapeutic range of dosage may lie close to toxic levels. Hospitalized patients are typically managed by more than one team of health care specialists, and the interventions of one team may conflict with the interventions and plans of another team. This potential for conflicting therapies requires that nurses carefully scrutinize plans of care by different medical consultants to ensure that they are compatible and consistent with the general medical consensus on every patient's diagnosis, plan of treatment, and nursing care.

As noted, nurses are present 24 hours a day with patients, and consequently play a crucial role in evaluating patients' responses to therapies and assessing changes in their patients' clinical conditions. This role requires that nurses be sufficiently engaged with their patients and remain attentive to possible significant physical and emotional changes, as well as to the social circumstances surrounding patients' illnesses and recovery. Nurses speak of their need to know their patients' concerns and clinical situations (Tanner et al., 1993). All of this monitoring requires astute diagnostic skills and clinical judgment on the part of the nurse (see Chapter 5). However, this judgment cannot come into play if the nurse does not have the time to properly monitor patients' therapies and assess patients' responses to those therapies. Attentiveness over time is required to identify subtle changes in a patient's condition.

Effective patient care requires that nurses advocate for their patients' best interests. Although nurses have an interprofessional alignment with physicians' goals for treatment and plans of care, nurses have a moral obligation to be aligned first and foremost with their patients' concerns and well-being. For example, if a patient needs urgent medical attention at an inconvenient hour for the physician, the patient's needs must come first.

OVERLAPPING NURSING CONCERNS IN GOOD NURSING PRACTICE

The nurse's attentiveness, skills of engagement with patients and their families, and patient advocacy go hand in hand. These caring practices are at the heart of good nursing practice. The nurse who does not or cannot meet with the patient/family because of patient care delivery design and/or assignment cannot come to understand the patient's concerns, clinical condition, and treatment plan. Consequently these nurses will not be able to notice significant changes in the patient's condition and will not learn what the patient's goals are with regard to treatment and care. The nurse-patient relationship establishes certain conditions that make it possible for patients to disclose their concerns, fears, and discomforts. If the nurse is too rushed or too task oriented to notice what the patient/family is experiencing, then the level of disclosure on the part of the patient/family will be constrained. Likewise, the nurse's attunement and engagement with the patient allows the nurse to notice subtle changes in the patient's condition.

As noted earlier, a socially organized practice such as nursing has notions of good internal to the practice (MacIntyre, 1984). For example, *attentiveness,* not neglect, and *recognition practices,* not depersonalization, are notions of good internal to the practice of nursing. A nurse educated to be an excellent nurse can recognize, in most instances, good and poor nursing care, even though it would be impossible to formally list all of the precise behaviors and comportment of excellent nursing care.

LIMITS OF FORMALISM

In philosophy, the inability to make explicit or formal all elements of a social practice identifies the limits of formalism (Dreyfus, 1992, pp. 35-51; Dreyfus & Dreyfus, 1986). For example, in nursing identifying learning objectives leads to the recognition that each objective is linked to many contexts and behaviors and that it is impossible to make explicit all of the background knowledge and contexts associated with the complex learning objectives in nursing. Likewise, the practical knowledge embedded in the traditions of science cannot be made completely formal and explicit (Dunne, 1997; Kuhn, 1977; Lave & Wenger, 1991). Every complex social practice has a foreground of focused attention and a background of comportment, practical skills, and understanding of the social practice. Science and technology have extensive traditions of formalizing the reasoning and knowledge associated with scientific experiments. Consequently it can appear to the naïve scientific practitioner that thinking within a particular scientific discipline is restricted to what can be formalized. This creates a risk to patient safety because a safe health care system depends on the attentive, knowledgeable work of professionals who must observe and detect signs of risk and/or danger and changes in patients' clinical situations. For example, in patient safety work the goal is to limit the attentiveness required by practitioners so that the patient's safety is not entirely dependent on constant practitioner attentiveness. This is only useful to the extent that it is possible and effective. Whatever can be made more reliable through automation and information system reminders can indeed improve patient safety. However, it must be continually recognized that health care practices are underdetermined, open ended, and complex, thus limiting the effectiveness of the usual strategies of automation and routinization. For example, automated intravenous fluid pumps can provide more accurate rates of delivery of fluids and medications. These machines are equipped with valuable alarm systems, but these systems must be set according to particular patient parameters and danger points. The constant attentiveness of the nurse to the intravenous pump is minimized by effective alarm systems, but defective alarms or parameters set inappropriately may tempt the practitioner to ignore the alarm or render it less sensitive to changes in the flow rate. The human factor must be taken into account and technological devices co-designed to fit the needs for adequate, but not excessive, attentiveness on the part of the nurse.

The attentive nurse and other health care providers remain the patient's front line of defense. The nurse is at the sharp end of practice and is often the last chance for patient care error to be averted (Benner, Hooper-Kyriakidis, & Stannard, 1999; Benner, Tanner, & Chesla, 1996; Page, 2004). Systems engineering must be cognizant of the goals of good practice, the requirements for effective surveillance, and the use of technology by nurses and other knowledge workers. Knowledge work and knowledge workers (a term used by sociologists) refer to any worker who requires a formal education for their work, who works in a field that requires ongoing knowledge development in their practice, usually a professional.

In practice disciplines such as nursing and medicine, the ethos of the practice shapes and is shaped by relevant science. The development of knowledge occurs in science and in experiential learning that comes directly from engaging in practice. Practice is a way of knowing in its own right, in this nontechnological understanding of what constitutes a practice and practice responsibilities (Benner, Hooper-Kyriakidis, & Stannard, 1999; Dunne, 1997; Taylor, 1993).

ATTENTIVENESS AND SURVEILLANCE

Attentiveness and surveillance of patients constitute moral acts as well as skillful judgment about what needs to be monitored for a patient's condition. The skills of attentiveness and noticing patient problems are developed both in nursing school and over time in nursing practice. However, when the institutional conditions for surveillance and attentiveness are impeded because of inadequate staffing or excessive "paperwork," then professional levels of attentiveness and surveillance of patients are likely to break down. Nurses who find themselves in situations of unsafe levels of staffing or excessive paperwork must have institutional avenues to demand correction of the staffing or paperwork in order to protect the patient.

LACK OF ATTENTIVENESS

Lack of attentiveness can also occur when a practitioner does not know what needs to be known or observed, or when the nurse does not observe and remain attuned to what is happening with patients and staff because of poor staffing, unsafe patient care assignments, lack of nursing knowledge, or other reasons (Benner et al., 2002). Inattentiveness to the point of patient neglect or abandonment is more than simply not paying attention and is as much a part of unprofessional conduct as fraudulent documentation or covering up a medication error.

Disruption of the nurse's attentiveness to patients is a barrier to quality nursing care and may prohibit the achievement of standards of nursing practice. Consequently lack of attentiveness, monitoring, and surveillance of patients may be grounds for reporting lack of attentiveness or surveillance to the state board of nursing for disciplinary action by the board. Occasionally nurses violate standards of good practice by leaving the patient care unit without notifying their colleagues and arranging adequate coverage for their patients; a just culture (Marx, 2001) calls for strict adherence to this minimal standard of professional responsibility. However, lack of surveillance is often due to miscommunication and conflict within a health care team or constant interruptions. Some hospitals have begun to use interventions to avoid interruptions of nurses during periods when they are administering medications. Nurses wear an apron signaling that they are carefully administering medications and should not be interrupted if at all possible. Of course, it takes cooperation and consensus among the health care team to change habits of interruption and make this work. A board of nursing looks carefully at the environmental, social, and personal causes of inattentiveness. Lack of nurse attentiveness is often associated with poor workload design or management. However, where patient surveillance is possible, it may be hindered by a lack of sufficient quality of engagement and interest in patient care on the part of the nurse.

In and of itself, a single incident of inattentiveness may not be a reportable offense to a board of nursing and may not even violate the laws regulating the practice of nursing. However, a detected pattern of inattentiveness may reveal that a nurse is practicing below the standard of professional practice or that some systems issues exist within the facility that impede or prevent the nurse's attentiveness to the patient's needs. A health care institution that does not plan for enough staff nurses to adequately monitor and pay attention to the patient's changing clinical condition or to patient responses to therapy, places patients and the nurses responsible for these patients at grave risk. Adequate monitoring of patients was identified as a greater problem in long-term care facilities, which are often understaffed, in our pilot work using the TERCAP® instrument.

The causes of deleterious consequences stemming from lack of attention and surveillance are difficult to identify. In the most obvious cases, if a patient has not been monitored or even seen by a nurse for more than 2 hours, the first undetected problem usually results from a lack of surveillance and monitoring rather than errors of clinical judgment. One cannot make good clinical judgments in the absence of attentiveness and monitoring of the patient.

The nurse, the team, the system, or a combination of the three may be complicit in lack of attentiveness and monitoring of patients. Ultimately, it is the responsibility of the nursing profession and institutions of health care to require the institutional possibility of monitoring patients' physiologic states, responses to therapies, and patient/family concerns.

When inattentiveness or a lapse of attention to subtle changes regarding a patient's condition occurs within the health care setting, an assessment and evaluation is needed to determine the reason for the occurrence. Consideration should be given to nursing issues related to a nurse being fatigued, being too busy, feeling overwhelmed, experiencing personal problems, or lacking necessary knowledge, skills, or abilities. The IOM report (Page, 2004) stated that the effects of fatigue include a lapse of attention to detail and can compromise one's problem-solving abilities. These factors along with poor staffing and workload design generate a culture that produces devastating effects on the possibility for attentive patient care.

The American Nurses Association (ANA) Code of Ethics for Nurses With Interpretative Statements (2001) identifies the responsibilities and duties for nurses. Provision 4 of the ANA Code states, "The nurse is responsible and accountable for individual nursing practice and determines the appropriate delegation of tasks consistent with the nurse's obligation to provide optimum patient care" (p. 16). Adhering to this particular provision of the ANA Code of Ethics requires critical thinking skills and making appropriate clinical judgments. Sound clinical judgment results from information produced through the design of safe and efficacious monitoring and surveillance of patients.

CHALLENGES

The challenge of providing public protection and safety with the provision of high-quality, cost-effective, and readily available and accessible nursing care is central to the mission of the nursing profession and the health care institutions that employ nurses. Every licensed nurse is required to adhere to his/her licensing board's scope of practice and is held accountable to his/her particular state board of nursing's nurse practice act. Likewise, nurses must be accountable for their nursing performance and actions in accordance with the minimal established standards of nursing practice. When the institutional conditions such as staffing and patient assignment make it impossible to live up to the Nursing Code of Ethics, the nurse is accountable for reporting such conditions.

LEGAL AND ETHICAL CHALLENGES

Nurses have a legal and ethical obligation to assess, plan, implement, and evaluate the care patients need. A nurse who does not access a patient or who is inattentive to the patient will be unable to implement the appropriate plan of care and therapeutic interventions necessary for that patient. The challenging and fast-paced world of health care has created additional needs for nurses within the health care setting. Nurses cannot individually overcome workplace demands and structures that disrupt attentiveness. Nurses need time to listen to their patients and to their staff. They are the eyes and ears for the patient. Patient safety depends on strategies and processes that are the result of collaborative efforts from the individual, the team, and the system that allows the nurse to pay attention to the subtle symptoms of a patient's condition, as well as to respond appropriately and in a timely manner.

Being observant of patients' needs can be as simple as checking the patency of a patient's IV or as complicated as detecting critical signs and symptoms of a patient's worsening condition. *Lack of attentiveness* indicates a lack of monitoring of therapies and patient responses on the part of the nurse and can result in serious injuries for the patient, even death (Benner, Hooper-Kyriakidis, & Stannard, 1999; Benner et al., 2002). As noted earlier, nursing errors can occur as a result of several factors. These include a lack of attentiveness due to increased workload, short staffing, failure to detect substandard care, lack of effective monitoring for an unsafe period of time, and failure to recognize an error.

Age-related factors, the mental status of a patient, cultural bearings, language deficits, and cognitive or functional abilities require even more attentiveness on the part of the nurse. Therefore nurses must have the moral agency, the professional responsibility, and the ethical duty to be attentive to their patients. Faulty supervision and the lack of appropriate staffing may be the underlying causes of an undetected critical patient condition when the nurse is overwhelmed with other patients or non-nursing duties. Given those factors, it is important to be responsible and declare one's unwillingness to work in that environment and setting but continue to do work on the particular shift where the need for nursing care is urgent and there are no additional nurses available. During a patient crisis, the system must be flexible and responsive enough to provide backup care for the nurse's other patients. Nurses must be able to see the overall situation, not just the one in front of them. Efforts to create a culture of safety in the health care environment include the ability to detect high-risk situations and the capacity to respond before an error or adverse event occurs.

RECOMMENDATIONS TO INCREASE ATTENTIVENESS/ SURVEILLANCE

On the basis of the above description of the role of nursing attentiveness, surveillance, and monitoring, health care teams and health care systems are advised to:

1. Provide education and communication regarding early identification and assessment of critical elements in each patient's monitoring and surveillance plan.
2. Encourage ongoing communication efforts, i.e., conduct hourly check-ins with team members, and report critical changes in patients' vital signs and physiologic states to the charge nurse and those at supervisory levels.
3. Prioritize the work as a team, helping those individuals who may have difficulty prioritizing needs in patients and in patient conditions with which they are unfamiliar or inexperienced.
4. Ensure the delegation of nursing interventions and the supervision of this delegation function.
5. Encourage cross-monitoring of work performance of health care team members.
6. Encourage input and collaboration from unlicensed assistive persons, staff nurses, management, leadership, and others on the health care team.
7. Engage the individual nurse, the team, and the system in identifying processes and strategies to create an attentive work environment.
8. Create a system of adequate attentiveness of patients while the nurse is on lunch and coffee breaks, and when a nurse needs a short break for excessive fatigue and sleepiness.
9. Design shift rotations with as much restorative time off as feasible.
10. Consult with nurses and counsel them on sleep hygiene.
11. Create an automated fast alert system such as a "computerized simple alert system "to supervisory personnel for increased acuity and or instability of the patient's condition on each nurse's patient care assignment. The supervisory response would be stipulated to reevaluate the adequacy of staffing and patient placement.
12. Create Fast Response Teams to respond to emergency situations and ensure that those teams monitor the care of the rest of the patients on the unit during a crisis.

HISTORICAL CASE STUDY #1: When Attentiveness and Surveillance Break Down

HISTORY

Mr. Harry Stewart was a resident who lived in a cottage on the grounds of a residential care facility. He required total nursing care as he was not able to bathe or dress himself. A patient care incident occurred at the cottage where it was discovered that a nurse was found to be negligent when she left Mr. Stewart in a bathtub unattended, and he was later found unconscious and pronounced dead on arrival (DOA) at an area hospital.

THE NURSE'S STORY

Ms. Mary Manning, a licensed practical nurse, was working the evening shift at the facility and had 40 residents assigned to her. These residents lived in various cottages on the facility grounds. Practical Nurse Manning went into one particular cottage to administer the scheduled 8:00 PM medications to the residents. She did not see Mr. Stewart when she entered his room. She moved to the bathroom and observed Mr. Stewart soaking in the bathtub. Practical Nurse Manning spoke with Mr. Stewart; he was alert, responsive, and talkative. She gave him his prescribed medications and proceeded to the living quarters of the cottage and approached the developmental assistant, Mr. Mark Randolph, who was assigned to this particular cottage. Practical Nurse Manning asked why Mr. Stewart was bathing unattended. Developmental Assistant Randolph replied that the other developmental assistant was out of the building and it was very busy that evening. Practical Nurse Manning completed the medication administration in that cottage and then left the building.

After leaving the cottage, Practical Nurse Manning returned to the office where she started her paperwork. Approximately one hour later, at 9:00 PM, she received a telephone call from Mr. Randolph who reported that he had found Mr. Stewart unconscious in the bathtub and thought Mr. Stewart had had a seizure and that he was dead. Practical Nurse Manning and her supervisor responded to the call, and on arrival they were directed to Mr. Stewart's bedroom.

Practical Nurse Manning reported that Developmental Assistant Randolph had removed Mr. Stewart from the bathtub and placed him on his bed. He said he had initially placed Mr. Stewart on the floor and started to administer CPR. Staff's efforts to resuscitate Mr. Stewart were unsuccessful. Emergency Medical Service personnel arrived within a short time, and Mr. Stewart was taken to the local hospital where he was pronounced dead.

Practical Nurse Manning reported that she asked Developmental Assistant Randolph if Mr. Stewart was supposed to be in the bathtub unattended. The response was that Mr. Stewart could not take care of himself and needed assistance at all times. Developmental Assistant Randolph went on to say that it was extremely busy that evening, and there was only one developmental assistant in the cottage to care for the clients and there was no possible way to provide assistance to every resident in the cottage. Developmental Assistant Randolph expressed concerns about being understaffed in addition to having a heavy workload, making it necessary to leave residents unattended at times in order to get his work done.

INTERVIEWS WITH WITNESSES

Staff members were fully aware that Mr. Stewart was totally dependent on nursing care and was not to be left unattended. Practical Nurse Manning stated that when she observed Mr. Stewart was unattended in the bathtub, it was her responsibility to take corrective action; however, instead, she gave Mr. Stewart his medications and left him alone in the bathtub. The facility reported that the only policy in place regarding leaving residents unattended in the bathtub addressed patients who might harm themselves and thus were not to be left unattended.

Authorities conducted an internal investigation and found that Practical Nurse Manning and other staff members failed to provide reasonable and necessary services to Mr. Stewart. The internal investigation concluded that Practical Nurse Manning and Developmental Assistant Randolph, the person in charge of Mr. Stewart, violated the facility's policies regarding the matter. Both were terminated from the employment setting as a result of the investigation by the facility and for reasons of neglect and negligence.

CASE ANALYSIS

Individual and team issues were both identified in this tragic case and resulted in lack of attentiveness by the nursing staff. The developmental assistant had the responsibility to provide safe patient care to all patients, and this was accomplished by communicating through the proper chain of command the need for additional help. The nurse in charge had the responsibility to act when she became aware of the fact that there was unsafe care being delivered to the patient. In fact, the licensed practical nurse is indeed at fault for failing to monitor her staff's performance. In addition, a question is raised: Was she simply doing her job of routinely administering medications without observing or assessing any of the patients' conditions? It appears that critical thinking and sound clinical judgment were absent when she saw Mr. Stewart in the bathtub alone. The patient records indicated that the patient required total nursing care. This fact, in itself, is evidence enough that the patient never should have been left alone in the bathtub. In this instance, two staff members understood this constraint, observed the patient unattended in the bathtub, and failed to assist him. Nurses are charged with the responsibility of providing safe patient care to all patients. Along with that responsibility is the expectation that attentiveness and surveillance will occur in order to maintain safe patient care.

HISTORICAL CASE STUDY #2: Attentiveness and Surveillance

THE IMPORTANCE OF CROSS-MONITORING TEAM MEMBERS' PERFORMANCES

HISTORY

This case involved three shifts of nurses over a 24-hour period working in a long-term care (LTC) facility. The facility included three separate units with 40 beds per unit. A licensed practical nurse charge nurse was assigned to each unit. One registered nurse supervisor was responsible per shift for the oversight of all three units.

Ms. Kathy Chin had been admitted to the LTC facility in October with heart failure, bipolar disorder with depression, constipation, history of gastrointestinal bleed, glaucoma, and discomfort. She required total care and was not able to effectively express her needs to the LTC staff. In January she had a bowel impaction, and Fleet enemas were administered. She was discovered unresponsive in her room the next afternoon and was transported to the hospital. Blood work revealed that she had a urinary tract infection. She was administered antibiotics and discharged back to the LTC facility.

Six weeks later, Ms. Chin had another episode of constipation. The day shift Nurse Supervisor, Ms. Angela Guilarte, notified Ms. Chin's physician, Dr. Brian Fisher. Dr. Fisher ordered an x-ray of Ms. Chin's abdomen, and it revealed severe constipation with fecal impaction. Dr. Fisher ordered clear liquids only and "Fleet enemas until clear." This was the same regime that was previously ordered and administered to Ms. Chin in January.

A licensed practical nurse, Ms. Margaret Reyes, took the order by telephone, notified day shift Nurse Supervisor Guilarte, documented the order in Ms. Chin's chart, as originally received from Dr. Fisher, and on the medication administration record [MAR] "enemas continuously until clear." Practical Nurse Reyes, who received the order for "Fleet enemas until clear," questioned the order and discussed it with Nurse Supervisor Guilarte. They determined that the enemas should be administered every 3 hours until the return was clear but did not clarify this with Dr. Fisher or pass this information on to the next shift.

The enemas were administered over a 12-hour period by three licensed practical nurses working various shifts. Again Ms. Chin was found unresponsive, and she was transferred to the hospital where she died 6 hours after admission.

THE NURSE'S STORY

I came to work early that evening and was told that the licensed practical charge nurse for one of the units had called in sick. I realized that I would have to cover the patients for the licensed practical nurse as well as provide supervision for the other two units. I received a short verbal report from Ms. Zellner, the evening shift registered nurse supervisor, who reported Ms. Chin's bowel impaction and the order to administer Fleet enemas until clear. I was told that Ms. Chin had been given three enemas prior to my shift.

It didn't occur to me that I should assess Ms. Chin and review her orders. I started administering the medications on the unit I was covering for the absent licensed practical nurse. About 3:00 AM, Ms. Mary Pellagros, a licensed practical nurse assigned to Ms. Chin, came to me and said she did not feel comfortable with the order for Fleet enemas until clear. Ms. Chin's blood pressure was 70/56, and eight enemas had been administered. She asked if the order should be changed. I told her to call Dr. Fisher. I also told Practical Nurse Pellagros to ask if we should start an IV for fluid replacement and draw stat labs to check her electrolytes. I did not assess Ms. Chin as I trusted Ms. Salamino to follow through.

Practical Nurse Pellagros later told me that Dr. Fisher repeated his order for "Fleet enemas until clear" and "reluctantly gave an order for an IV." Dr. Fisher refused to order *stat labs*. I didn't ask Practical Nurse Pellagros if she had informed Dr. Fisher of the number of enemas that had been administered (eight). It took several hours for the IV fluid and pump to be delivered to the facility. I went to Ms. Chin's room and started the IV. I did not conduct an assessment, but Ms. Chin was responsive. At the end of the shift, I reported off to the Shift Supervisor Guilarte and told her about the new orders that were obtained during the night. I did not report the number of enemas given on the night shift (eight plus four), and I did not check to see if vital signs had been documented during the night shift.

It is my understanding that the day shift administered three more enemas to Ms. Chin after which, at 1:00 PM, she was found to be unresponsive. She was then transferred to the hospital. I trusted Practical Nurse Pellagros to provide the care Ms. Chin required. Nurse Pellagros called Dr. Fisher and carried out his orders. I didn't believe it was my responsibility to challenge a physician's order, and I didn't believe I should call my supervisor, the Director of Nursing, in the middle of the night.

INTERVIEWS WITH WITNESSES

All staff members who participated in or were present during the period of time the enemas were given were fully aware of Ms. Chin's history and the outcome she experienced with the first bowel impaction she had in January. None of the staff members were aware of the number of enemas that were administered during the second episode over the 12-hour time frame, after the order was received from the physician.

Dr. Fisher stated that Practical Nurse Pellagros called him during the night and questioned the order for enemas until clear but did not tell him how many enemas had actually been administered. He refused to clarify the order and believed the order was appropriate as he had given it. He said Practical Nurse Pellagros should have used her "common sense and not administered that many." We recommend the use of the SBAR communication approach, which provides the standard framework for conveying key information. (The acronym stands for Situation—a brief statement of the problem; Background relevant for the situation at hand; Assessment—summary of what the clinician believes is the underlying cause and its severity; and Recommendation—what is needed to resolve the situation [Pope, Rodzen, & Gross, 2008].)

CASE ANALYSIS

This case demonstrates the fatal outcome that emerged when nurses did not recognize the importance of continuous attentiveness and surveillance when providing what is perceived to be routine care. Bowel care in a long-term care facility is a part of most residents' care plans and is competently provided by licensed practical nurses, and sometimes by unlicensed assistive personnel.

The registered nurse supervisor did not recognize her responsibility to intervene when the licensed practical nurse came to her with questions about the physician's order and reported that the patient's blood pressure was low. The registered nurse did not fully assess the situation or the patient. She provided the licensed practical nurse with some suggestions, such as requesting an order from the physician for IV fluid replacement and a stat blood draw. She was aware that the patient's condition was declining but allowed the licensed practical nurse to continue to carry out an order that would endanger the patient. By not assessing the patient herself, she did not provide the input necessary to give the physician a clear picture of the patient's declining physical status and did not intervene when the physician continued to refuse to discuss further options for her care. The registered nurse did not contact her supervisor to obtain direction when she knew the physician's order was not appropriate. She did not check back with the licensed practical nurse and reassess the patient.

There were systems breakdowns as well as individual practice breakdowns that led to the patient's death. The LTC facility did not have a system in place to address short staffing when a licensed practical charge nurse was unavailable for work. This meant that the evening supervisor had to fill in for the absent licensed practical nurse and sacrificed the attention needed for supervisory functions during the shift. The environment provided by facility management did not encourage the registered nurse supervisor to contact the director of nursing with concerns regarding emerging issues during the night shift. The registered nurse supervisor did not understand her responsibility to assess the resident and provide adequate surveillance to ensure that the licensed practical nurse who was providing the direct care was meeting the patient's needs. The registered nurse did not initiate follow-up with the licensed practical nurse to ensure that the patient's status did not continue to decline. The registered nurse should have contacted the physician and challenged the order for "Fleet enemas until clear."

In this case, lack of attentiveness and surveillance and faulty intervention on the part of the registered nurse supervisor prevented the patient from receiving the interventions required for her declining physical condition. The registered nurse supervisor contributed to the patient's death with the inappropriate administration of the physician's faulty order. This cascade of errors could have been prevented if the registered nurse supervisor, who was aware of the patient's history, had identified her responsibility to provide attentive surveillance of this emerging and preventable situation.

SUMMARY

Monitoring and thoughtfully observing and responding to changes in a patient's clinical condition or concerns is a bedrock nursing function and skill. Attentiveness without engagement with the patient falls short as these extreme cases illustrate. Sleepiness, fatigue, and disengagement are all personal factors that influence the attentiveness required for effective monitoring and surveillance of patients. Poor staffing, a culture of low expectations, and an inadequate staff mix of professional nurses and unlicensed assistants are institutional factors that disrupt attentiveness. Patients who are somnolent, cognitively impaired, or have a decreased level of consciousness are at great risk when nursing surveillance and monitoring are below standard. Patients who cannot effectively call for help or articulate their needs depend on the attentiveness of nurses to protect them from the many threats to their safety while they are hospitalized.

References

Aiken, L. H., Clarke, S. P., Cheung, R. B., Sloane, D. M., & Silber, J. H. (2003). Educational levels of hospital nurses and surgical patient mortality. *Journal of the American Medical Association, 290*(12), 1617-1623.

Aiken, L. H., Clarke, S. P., Sloane, D. M., Sochalski, J., & Silber, J. H. (2002). Hospital nurse staffing and patient mortality, nurse burnout, and job dissatisfaction. *Journal of the American Medical Association, 288*(16), 1987-1993.

American Nurses Association (ANA). (2001). *Code of ethics for nurses with interpretative statements.* Washington, DC: ANA.

Benner, P., Hooper-Kyriakidis, P., & Stannard, D. (1999). *Clinical wisdom and interventions in critical care: A thinking-in-action approach.* Philadelphia: W.B. Saunders.

Benner, P., Sheets, V., Uris, P., Malloch, K., Schwed, K., & Jamison, D. (2002). Individual, practice, and system causes of errors in nursing: A taxonomy. *Journal of Nursing Administration, 32*(10), 509-523.

Benner, P., Tanner, C. A., & Chesla, C. A. (1996). *Expertise in nursing practice: Caring, clinical judgment and ethics.* New York: Springer.

Cho, S. K., Ketefian, S., Barkauskas, H., & Smith, D. G. (2003). The effects of nurse staffing on adverse events, morbidity, mortality and medical costs. *Nursing Research, 52*(2), 71-79.

Clarke, S. P., & Aiken, L. H. (2003). Failure to rescue. *American Journal of Nursing, 103* (1), 42-47.

Coffey, L. C., Skipper, J. K., Jr., & Jung, F. D. (1988). Nurses and shift work: Effects on job performance and job-related stress. *Journal of Advanced Nursing, 13*(2), 245-254.

Dreyfus, H. L. (1992). *What computers still can't do: A critique of artificial reason.* Cambridge, MA: Massachusetts Institute of Technology Press.

Dreyfus, H. L., & Dreyfus, S. E. (1986). *Mind over machine: The power of human intuition and expertise in the era of the computer.* New York: Free Press.

Dunne, J. (1997). *Back to the rough ground: Practical judgment and the lure of technique.* Notre Dame, IN: University of Notre Dame Press.

Kuhn, T. S. (1977). *The essential tension: Selected studies in scientific tradition and change.* Chicago: University of Chicago Press.

Lave, J., & Wenger, E. (1991). *Situated learning, legitimate peripheral perspectives: Learning in doing, social, cognitive and computational perspectives.* Cambridge: Cambridge University Press.

MacIntyre, A. (1984). *After virtue: A study in moral theory* (2nd ed.). Notre Dame, IN: University of Notre Dame Press.

Marx, D. (2001). *Patient safety and the "just culture": A primer for health care executives.* New York: Columbia University Press.

Maxfield, D., Grenny, J., McMillan, R., Patterson, K., & Switzler, A. (2005). Silence kills: The seven crucial conversations in health care. *VitalSmarts Industry Watch*. Available online at www.silencekills.com. Accessed October, 1, 2008.

Mitler, M. M., Carskadon, M. A., Czeisler, C. A., Dement, W. C., Dinges, D. F., & Graeber, R. C. (1988). Catastrophes, sleep, and public policy: consensus report. *Sleep*, *11*(1), 100-109.

Mustard, L. W. (2002). The culture of patient safety. *JONA's Healthcare Law, Ethics, and Regulation*, *4*(4), 111-115.

Needleman, J., Buerhaus, P., Mattke, S., Stewart, M., & Zelevinsky, K. (2002). Nurse-staffing levels and the quality of care in hospitals. *New England Journal of Medicine*, *346*(22), 1715-1722.

Page, A. (Ed.); Committee on the Work Environment for Nurses and Patient Safety, Institute of Medicine. (2004). *Keeping patients safe: Transforming the work environment of nurses*. Washington, D.C.: The National Academies Press.

Pope, B. B., Rodzen, L., & Spross, G. (2008). Raising the SBAR: how better communication improves patient outcomes. *Nursing*, *38*(3), 41-43.

Reason, J. T. (1990). *Human error*. New York: Cambridge University Press.

Rosekind, M. R., Gregory, K. B., Miller, D. L., Co, E. L., & Lebacqz, J. V. (1994). *Aircraft accident report: Uncontrolled collision with terrain*. American International Airways Flight 808, Douglas DC-8, N814CK, U.S. Naval Air Station, Guantanamo Bay, Cuba, August 18, 1993: National Transportation Safety Board.

Smith-Coggins, R., Howard, S. K., Mac, D. T., Wang, C., Kwan, S., Rosekind, M. R., et al (2006). Improving alertness and performance in emergency department physicians and nurses: the use of planned naps. *Annals of Emergency Medicine*, *48*(5), 596-604.

Smith-Coggins, R., Rosekind, M. R., Buccino, K. R., Dinges, D. F., & Moser, R. P. (1997). Rotating shiftwork schedules: can we enhance physician adaptation to night shifts? *Academic Emergency Medicine*, *4*(10), 951-961.

Smith-Coggins, R., Rosekind, M. R., Hurd, S., & Buccino, K. R. (1994). Relationship of day versus night sleep to physician performance and mood. *Annals of Emergency Medicine*, *24*(5), 928-934.

Tanner, C., Benner, P., Chesla, C., & Gordon, D. (1993). The phenomenology of knowing a patient. *Journal of Nursing Scholarship*, *25*(4), 273-280.

Taylor, C. (1993). Explanation and practical reason. In M. Nussbaum & A. Sen (Eds.), *The quality of life* (pp. 208-231). Oxford: Clarendon.

Ulrich, R., Quan, X., Zimring, C., Joseph, A., & Choudhary, R. (2004). *The role of the physical environment in the hospital of the 21st century: A once-in-a-lifetime opportunity*. Concord, CA: The Center for Health Design.

Weick, K. E., & Sutcliff, K. M. (2001). *Managing the unexpected: Assuring high performance in an age of complexity*. San Francisco: Jossey-Bass.

Wylie, C., Schultz, T., Miller, J., Mitler, M., & Mackie, R. (1996). *Commercial motor vehicle driver fatigue and alertness study*. FHWA Report number: FHWA-MC-97-001, TC Report Number TP12876E. Montreal, Canada: Transportation Development Center. Prepared for the Federal Highway Administration, U.S. Department of Transportation; Trucking Research Institute, American Trucking Associations Foundation; and the Transportation Development Centre, Safety and Security, Transport Canada.

5

Practice Breakdown: Clinical Reasoning or Judgment

Patricia Benner ◆ *Vicki Goettsche* ◆ *Karla Bitz*

Chapter Outline

Clinical reasoning is a basic requirement for all health care workers. The understanding and distinctiveness of this category has evolved over the course of the practice breakdown work. Initially this category was labeled, not surprisingly, as *clinical judgment*. However, the lack of conceptual clarity and discreteness became apparent as discussion and uses continued regarding the data collection instruments in pilot cases.

The Practice Breakdown Advisory Panel (PBAP) recognized that clinical judgment was involved in most of the practice breakdown categories and was difficult to isolate to a single category. The challenge was to specify the infrastructure or the defined process within clinical judgment—namely, the role of perceptual acuity and the ability to assess and determine the appropriate course of action based on that perception. Clinical reasoning came to be identified as nurses' reasoning about titration of medications such as vasopressors to keep patients within certain hemodynamic parameters. The most dynamic area of clinical reasoning in current nursing practice concerns reasoning across time about patients' responses to therapies. Often the margin between a therapeutic response and an overtreatment or undertreatment or an untoward effect is narrow and varies among patients. For example, titrating doses of pain medication to adequately relieve pain for particular patients is highly variable and requires astute clinical reasoning about the patient's responses over time.

After much dialogue, members determined that the label of clinical judgment did not convey the highly skilled and complex work of nursing. To address this concern, the category was named "diagnostic discernment" and then finally changed to "clinical reasoning" to more accurately identify the work of nurses and to further distinguish this dimension of clinical judgment.

Nurses engage in diagnostic discernment or clinical reasoning in which multiple influences are present. Good clinical reasoning requires perceptual acuity, the skills of attentiveness and involvement, and the skills of moral agency and advocacy. In turn, these skills are mediated through challenged work environments that must contend with the nursing shortages and the forces of a competitive marketplace.

DIAGNOSTIC DISCERNMENT AND PERCEPTUAL ACUITY

Perceptual awareness is the skill of seeing and noticing; it requires skillful engagement, both with problems and persons. Skills of recognition, visual discrimination, and comparative distinctions are implied. This definition is from Benner, Hooper-Kyriakidis, & Stannard (1999) and the following presentation draws heavily on their work.

Identifying and solving problems is essential to effective and safe nursing practice. However, effective problem solving depends on perceptual acuity and recognizing when a problem is critical and needs assessment and intervention. If a nurse's assignment does not permit sufficient attentiveness and monitoring of the patient, the nurse will not have an opportunity to exercise good clinical judgment. If a nurse does not understand a patient's clinical condition and treatment, then the patient's problems may be framed or defined in misguiding ways that may cause the nurse to overlook significant signs and symptoms. Thus attentiveness is essential for good nursing practice. As a moral art, attentiveness requires the emotional skills of openness and responsiveness (Vetleson, 1994). A lack of attentiveness and engagement with the patient's situation results in a nurse's lack of a good grasp of the situation. If work design and nurse staffing do not allow sufficient time for observing and assessing the patient, then the nurse will be handicapped in gaining a good clinical understanding of the patient's clinical condition.

Sometimes the definition of a problem makes it unsolvable, and redefining or reframing the problem can create new options. Problem identification (which problem[s] does the clinician perceive and seek to solve) requires perceptual acuity. One *may* have the appropriate intellectual understanding of particular clinical entities and ethical issues but may not have the perceptual acuity to recognize when these issues are at stake in actual situations. Perceptual acuity is linked to emotional engagement with the problem and interpersonal engagement with patients and families (Benner & Wrubel, 1982). Patients and families will choose to disclose their fears and concerns only if there seems to be sufficient time and interest on the part of the nurse.

Perception requires skillful engagement both with the problem and the person(s). Perceptual acuity is much less studied than judgment, yet one can only make judgments about what is perceived (Vetleson, 1994). The skills of problem engagement and interpersonal involvement require experiential learning. For example, clinicians talk about problems of overidentifying with the patient and becoming flooded with feelings. It is equally a problem to wall off feelings so that the possibilities of attunement are blunted or shut down. The beginning nurse can feel a generalized anxiety over the demands of learning or the fear of making errors. At this beginning stage, dampening emotional responses can lower anxiety and improve performance. But with the gaining of skilled know-how and good clinical judgment, emotional responses can become more differentiated. The practitioner begins to feel comfortable and "at home" in familiar situations and uneasy in situations that are unfamiliar. This differentiated emotional response is the beginning of gaining a sense of salience and developing attunement to the situation. At the competent stage, clinical learners can safely pay attention to vague or global emotional responses as a sign that they do not fully understand a situation. This global understanding of the clinical situation is at the heart of practical clinical reasoning that we call *clinical grasp* (Benner, Hooper-Kyriakidis, & Stannard, 1999). At the competent level of skill acquisition, nurses have a developing sense of *when* they do or do not have a good clinical grasp of the situation. This emotional sense is crucial to early problem search and identification. Perceptual acuity and an acute clinical grasp of the situation are the sources of discovery and early warnings of changes in patients.

Traditionally, emotion has been seen as the opposite of cognition and rationality. But increasingly it is recognized that emotions play a key role in perception and even act as a moral compass in learning a practice (Benner, Tanner, & Chesla, 1996; Dreyfus, Dreyfus, & Benner, 1996). For example, at the competent stage, clinical learners feel "good" when they perform well and when they take the risks inherent in making sound clinical judgments. Nurses at this level feel disappointment and regret when an error in judgment causes a patient to suffer a negative outcome (Dreyfus & Dreyfus, 1986). These are essential aesthetic and ethical responses that guide the development of perceptual acuity and problem identification. And it is the ongoing background sense of whether the nurse has a good grasp of a clinical situation or whether the situation is ambiguous and puzzling that guides problem recognition and clarification.

DIAGNOSTIC DISCERNMENT AND ATTENTIVENESS

Interpersonal engagement is not synonymous with problem engagement, although the two are linked. Bearing witness to another's distress can cause anxiety, and nurses may distance themselves for their own emotional protection. If nurses selectively attend to *some* problems more than others, such as attending to a patient's dysrhythmias or cardiac output, they may not be able to engage with the patient's overall clinical situation. They must learn to carry out comprehensive assessment of the patient's changes over time.

Anxiety can disrupt attentiveness and helping relationships. Extreme disengagement may prevent the nurse from experiencing personal responsibility and agency in a clinical situation (Rubin, 1996). Thus attentiveness as disrupted by system constraints, such as low nurse-to-patient staffing ratios, may prevent sufficient nurse-patient contact to ensure attentiveness. It cannot be considered an error of "clinical judgment" if system constraints have prevented the nurse from having sufficient contact with a patient to make an adequate assessment of the patient's condition. For reasoning-in-transition (or practical clinical reasoning) to occur, the nurse must use the interpersonal skills of engaging with the clinical and human situation at hand but he/she must also have the opportunity to interact with the patient. The relational skills of listening to and clarifying the patient's concern create effective disclosure spaces for understanding the patient's situation and needs.

Thus attentiveness is related to skills of involvement or engagement. Attentiveness and skills of involvement require the imperative of an open and attentive engagement with a clinical situation or problem and the skill of applying the right kinds and amounts of interpersonal engagement with patients and their families (Benner, Hooper-Kyriakidis, & Stannard, 1999).

CASE STUDY—BEWARE: One Emergency May Hide Another!

A hospital submitted a report to the State Board of Nursing reporting that an RN had been terminated after the death of a patient following surgery for a tubal pregnancy.

THE NURSE'S STORY—SALLY SIMMS, RN

I had worked the medical-surgical units at the General Hospital ever since graduating from my nursing program 4 years before. This was the worst night, the worst shift, of my nursing career.

I was assigned to care for eight patients that night, which is not an unusual number of patients, but they all were either fresh post-ops or so very sick. Four patients had just had surgery that day. One patient was on a dopamine drip to maintain his blood pressure, so he needed frequent monitoring. One patient was suspected to have meningitis, one patient had pneumonia, and a patient with suspected histoplasmosis completed my assignment.

One of my post-op patients was Betty Smith, a young woman in her early thirties who had laparoscopic surgery late in the day. She had been transferred from the recovery room late in the evening shift and was very uncomfortable when I first made my rounds. At 12:05 AM, I called Betty's physician because she was vomiting and thrashing in bed. Per his order, I medicated the patient with Phenergan.

The next time I checked on Betty, she seemed to be more comfortable, but I realized that her IV had infiltrated. I was really overwhelmed with meeting the needs of all my patients, so I asked Joan Jones, the charge nurse, to restart Betty's IV. It was about 2:00 AM when Nurse Joan restarted the IV.

I had been able to pretty much stay on top of everything at that point in the shift, and by 2:30 AM I had assessed all my patients, given pain medications, and called four physicians to update them regarding their patients and for various orders. I thought things were settling down. I thought wrong.

Mrs. Holmes, the patient with histoplasmosis, seemed a bit off from when I had cared for her the previous two nights. Mrs. Holmes' vital signs were unstable and her O_2 saturation was only 80%. I notified her physician and he ordered stat arterial blood gases. The lab called with the results, and they were alarming. Mrs. Homes was losing ground, and her physician ordered us to transfer her to the ICU. I was preoccupied with accomplishing the transfer and accompanied Mrs. Holmes to the unit. I returned from the ICU at about 3:50 AM.

On my return, I first checked the patient who was on dopamine, medicated another patient for pain, and did visual checks on the rest of the patients who all seemed to be sleeping. I began my charting.

At 6:05 AM, I went to start IV antibiotics on Betty's roommate, and to my horror discovered Betty was not breathing. I called the code. The first time I discovered that Betty had had a low blood pressure and elevated pulse was when I checked the vital signs sheet when the ER physician (who responded to the code) asked how Betty's vital signs had been during the shift. The nurse's aide who was assigned to monitor Betty had not informed me, and I had not checked the vital signs sheet.

It was such a terrible night; I was so busy with the transfer and caring for the other patients. Betty just had an outpatient procedure; if she had been earlier on the surgical schedule, they would have sent her home. I did not physically check her vital signs, and the aide did not report the elevated pulse and low blood pressure. I depended on the aide—my mistake. I know I was responsible.

I was terminated from employment and reported to the board of nursing. I have taken myself out of nursing; something died in me when I found my patient.

EMPLOYMENT EVALUATIONS

An evaluation conducted a few weeks before the incident showed mostly good ratings (11) with three excellent ratings. The hospital would consider reemployment if Ms. Simms improved her critical thinking skills.

PATIENT MEDICAL RECORD

Surgery Notes—Laparoscopy to remove unruptured ectopic pregnancy from distal portion of the fimbriae with estimated blood loss of 150 cc, three references to homeostasis, two references to cautery, patient ". . . to recovery room in excellent condition."

Recovery Room Nurse's Notes—In recovery 2110 to 2300, initial post-op flow sheet noted at 2210 BP 124/74, pulse 94; at 2225 BP 123/65; at 2240 BP 107/85, pulse 123. Assessment signed at 2220 "abdomen distended with few faint bowel sounds ... patient shivering, c/o [complained of] abdominal pain, medicated ×3 [three times] with IVP Demerol, total of 50 mg. Patient awake, three dressings dry. No c/o N/V/D." [No complaints of nausea, vomiting or diarrhea.]

Medication Record—Patient received Demerol 50 mg. with 25 mg Phenergan IM at 2215 and 0200.

Cardiopulmonary Resuscitation Record—Compressions noted at 6:08 AM. [RN had initiated code at 5:55 AM], MD arrived at 6:15 AM, patient intubated at 6:20 AM, patient administered atropine ×3, Eppy [epinephrine] ×5 [five times], bicarbonate [of sodium] ×2 [two times]. Pacemaker never captured. Patient never had return of spontaneous pulses and pronounced dead at 6:38 AM.

Death Certificate—Immediate cause of death was hemoperitoneum due to postoperative hemorrhage of placental tissues after salpingotomy for a right tubal ectopic pregnancy.

BOARD ACTION

Ms. Simms entered into a consent agreement with the board of nursing, admitting that her conduct constituted a failure to practice in accordance with acceptable and prevailing standards of safe nursing care. Nursing standards cited were failure to assess and document the health status of the patient, failure to provide ongoing patient monitoring, and failure to communicate appropriately with members of the health care team.

Ms. Simms' license was probated with stayed suspension for 2 years, with requirements for successful completion of ordered education including an advanced assessment course at an educational/collegiate institution, continuing education hours in risk management/legal issues in nursing (in addition to continuing education hours required for license renewal). Order noted RN's voluntary evaluation by a mental health care professional and her compliance with all aspects of the treatment plan. Other terms included quarterly reports from nursing employer and self-reports. Ms. Simms was required to appear in person (as requested) for an interview with the Board or a board-designated representative.

COMMENTARY

This case example illustrates a cascade of clinical events that caused errors in clinical judgment, all of which are related to work overload and consequent lack of surveillance and monitoring of the patient. Nurse Simms made faulty assumptions that the young patient with a tubal pregnancy was her least acute patient. Of course the patient is the primary victim, but Nurse Simms also suffered greatly from this tragic incident, which was precipitated by a collection of untoward events and work overload. The following TERCAP® categories under "Inadequate Clinical Judgment" are appropriate:

Clinical implications of signs, symptoms, and/or interventions not recognized: The abdominal pain was extreme for the procedure and was most likely related to internal hemorrhage.

Clinical implications of signs, symptoms, and/or interventions misinterpreted: The nurse assumed that the primary problem was nausea and vomiting. Other vital signs and symptoms were ignored.

Lack of appropriate priorities: In this case there were at least three competing high-priority situations occurring at once.

Poor judgment in delegation and the supervision of other staff members: Delegation and supervision were problems on several levels. The charge nurse and supervisor failed to provide appropriate support for the RN with a patient in a full-blown crisis. The nurse gave the nurse's aide faulty supervision in not requesting full vital signs at 5:00 AM.

Inappropriate acceptance of assignment or delegation beyond the nurse's knowledge, skills, and abilities (given the critical and unstable condition of the eight patients): Eight patients were too many patients to care for given the critical acuity of these particular eight patients. Backup support should have been requested and/or just sent when one patient went into crisis. The nursing supervisor is mistaken in waiting for reports only as a means of knowing what is needed, especially when a patient crisis arises.

CLARIFYING CONCEPTS

During the initial examination of many of the study cases, poor clinical judgment was identified as the cause of the practice breakdown. Often, however, the cause for the practice breakdown was lack of attentiveness. Nurses were not able to begin to engage in a clinical situation and begin to use their clinical judgment because of staffing shortages and competing high priorities among patients. Recommendations to remediate nurse clinical judgment skills in such situations would be nonproductive. Also, a unit can have a very hectic day with more patients admitted than usual, or more patient crises than usual, causing many disruptions to many nurses' work on the unit. Nurses are called to watch over patients for other nurses and may not have a good grasp of the patient's ongoing clinical condition and needs. Thus, as discussed in Chapter 4, the issue of attentiveness needs to be addressed in ways that allow the nurse adequate time for attentiveness or awareness of the clinical situation to prevent practice breakdown. If the unit is unusually pressed, short staffed, or the nurse is interrupted frequently because of a heavy workload, a patient in crisis, or new patient admissions, the root cause of the problem may not be clinical reasoning but a system-induced lack of adequate patient monitoring.

All nursing actions contain within them some form of judgment. For the purposes of TERCAP classification of nursing practice breakdown, we are using a restricted definition of *clinical reasoning* (as described above) because we want to identify situations where knowledge and skill related to clinical judgment are absent or obsolete. In these instances the nurse misinterprets or makes a mistake in judgment about a patient's needs or concerns, *even though he/she has had the opportunity to observe the patient.* Common, routine interventions that are required for all patients should not be considered an issue or a problem of *clinical judgment,* since the primary problem is an omission of routine, standardized practice that requires knowledge. For example, although it is always poor judgment to omit preventive interventions, it is really not an issue of clinical reasoning about a particular patient to omit standard nursing procedures to avoid the hazards of mobility. Likewise, standard infection preventive measures require little latitude or room for judgment and should not be classified as clinical judgment.

Poor clinical judgment will impact the ability of the nurse to advocate for the patient, but if the nurse makes an appropriate clinical judgment but does not follow through with adequate advocacy for the patient, (e.g., calling the physician for an appropriate intervention), then the primary area of practice breakdown is Professional Responsibility and Patient Advocacy. Clinical judgment is always situated. Good clinical judgment requires the possibility of attentiveness. In the one clinical situation above, a nurse had an extremely heavy assignment with the same-day postsurgical patients, one of whom required a vasopressor to maintain his blood pressure. To complicate the situation further, another patient with histoplasmosis developed poor oxygen saturation and required an immediate transfer to the ICU. The transfer of the patient with poor oxygen saturation took the nurse away from the unit at a critical time for the patient after she had had a tubal pregnancy removed; she was now showing all the signs of a postoperative hemorrhage. As a result of information overload and poor backup support, the nurse did not receive or could not attend to the 30-year-old patient who was experiencing a postoperative hemorrhage and extreme pain.

There are human limits to the span of control and the ability to attend to multiple urgent and cognitively complex demands. Many system and practice breakdowns came together at the same time to create this tragic outcome of patient death. The nurse's aide was not appropriately respectful and attentive to the patient's requests to call her husband and her physician. The patient was labeled "whiny" and her complaints, as well as the patient's authority, were devalued and dismissed. The charge nurse did not adequately assess the nurse's workload. The supervisory practice in the hospital was substandard in that clinical supervisors did not proactively observe and supervise the unit's workload, changing conditions, and the nursing needs of the patients. Rather, supervisory staff waited until they received an explicit request for help from very busy nurses. There was no Fast Response Team to come to the unit. It may seem obvious that busy, overloaded nurses would automatically call for help, but there is little support for this assumption, because the nurse who is busy phoning physicians and carrying out emergency interventions may be so occupied with urgent, multiple demands that making one more phone call in the moment does not occur to him or her. If help is seldom provided when requested, it may also seem futile to take the time to call.

An intervention at the system level would be a predetermined "SOS" number that requires no explanation or rationale and that receives immediate supervisory attention. Such a signal would require an immediate, mandatory response from nursing supervisory staff, including the immediate nursing staff on the unit. Patients should be routinely given a supervisory number to call 24 hours a day, whenever they feel that their needs are not being adequately attended to on any nursing unit. In this situation, such a routine "fail-safe" backup strategy for patients could have possibly prevented this patient's death. The patient tried to call her husband for help, and she tried to call her physician. The patient did not imagine that there was any available help in the hospital because her requests were being ignored by the nurse's aide, and the busy registered nurse had little first-hand contact with the patient.

No doubt the nurse's information and task overload caused her to deviate from the professional standard of care of closely monitoring the patient's vital signs postoperatively, checking for potential hemorrhage, and assessing the patient's pain. In the context of two competing patients' urgent care needs, the nurse did not make a direct assessment of the postoperative patient's condition on receiving information from the nurse's aide about the patient's changing vital signs. The period of decreased surveillance and monitoring prevented adequate clinical observation, assessment, and thus detection of postoperative hemorrhage that, if recognized, would have saved this patient's life. In this instance, a critical lack of surveillance occurred during which time the nurse instructed the nurse's aide not to awaken the patient and check her vital signs at 5:00 AM. It is unknown whether the patient was indeed sleeping, unconscious, or dead at 5:00 AM. when the nurse's aide reported that the patient was sleeping quietly.

Good clinical reasoning requires knowledge about the patient's particular condition and therapies being used. Clinical reasoning also requires the ability to perceive and recognize changes in patients' clinical conditions and responses to ongoing therapy. Unlike scientific reasoning that can be established using formal criteria and decision points at prescribed points in time, clinical reasoning is ongoing about the particular in relation to the general. Clinical reasoning is reasoning across time, about the particular, through changes in the patient's condition and/or changes in the clinician's understanding of the patient's condition over time (Benner, Hooper-Kyriakidis, & Stannard, 1999).

Benner, Hooper-Kyriakidis, & Stannard (1999) state:

> Critical care nursing practice is intellectually and emotionally challenging because it requires quick judgments and responses to life-threatening conditions where there are narrow margins for error. Developing expertise in this practice requires experiential learning under pressure and "thinking-in-action" (thinking linked with action in ongoing situations) (p. 2).

The nurse's overload and focused concern for the patient whom she considered to be at greatest risk, clouded her thinking-in-action about her other patient's potential for hemorrhage, and therefore caused her to ignore warning signs of changes in the patient's condition.

Clinical judgment requires clinical reasoning across time about the particular. Clinical reasoning is very different from scientific reasoning in conducting clinical or bench research. Research uses formal criteria to develop "yes" and "no" judgments. Research is closer to a static, snapshot reasoning than clinical reasoning which, as noted, is reasoning across time about the particular through changes in the clinician's understanding or changes in the patient's condition.

> Nursing, like medicine, involves a rich, socially embedded, clinical know-how that encompasses perceptual skills, transitional understandings across time, and understanding of the particular in relation to the general. Clinical knowledge is a form of engaged reasoning that follows *modus operandi thinking* in relation to patients' and clinical populations' particular manifestations of disease, dysfunction, response to treatment, and recovery trajectories. Clinical knowledge is necessarily configurational, historical (by historical, we mean the immediate and long-term histories of particular patients and clinical populations), contextual, perceptual, and based upon knowledge gained in transitions...[Through articulation], clinical understanding becomes increasingly articulate and translatable at least by clinical examples, narratives, and puzzles encountered in practice (Benner, 1994, p. 139).

Clinical reasoning also requires engaged reasoning across time about the particular through changes in the patient's condition and changes in the clinician's understanding of the patient's situation (Benner, 1984, 2001). Aristotle called attention to practice or *praxis* that requires *phronesis,* something qualitatively distinct from *techne* (the know-how and skill of producing things). This was in addition to the narrower "rational calculation" or snapshot account of rationality handed down in the Cartesian tradition and captured in early Greek thought by Plato as *techne* or technique. A practice is a socially embedded form of knowledge that has notions of the good internal to the practice (Benner, 1984, 2001). Aristotle's example was that of a statesman who had to develop character, skilled know-how, practical reasoning, and comportment that included appropriate emotional responses and relationships. This contrast form of rationality and skill-based character called *phronesis* is similar to clinical judgment. A rational-technical mode, techne (sometimes called "rational technicality"), separates means and ends and focuses on achieving prespecified outcomes.

Rational technical thought is a powerful strategy for those areas of science and technology that can be standardized and made routine. But where clinical reasoning, relationship, perception (or noticing), timing, and skilled know-how are involved, more than techne or rational calculation is required. Guignon (1983) points out that separating means and outcomes often devalues or does violence to the means, especially where means and ends are closely interwoven. For example, it is not sensible to separate means and ends in birth, comfort, health promotion, or end-of-life care. In each of these caring practices, means and ends are in many ways not separable, since most often there are multiple means and ends at stake in any clinical encounter.

Caregiving relationships may open up possibilities or close them down. But even with the best intentions and comportment, the one cared for may not be able to respond to care. "Outcomes" in caregiving relationships are necessarily interdependent and mutual. Some types of influence are morally unacceptable. Manipulation, coercion, or misuse of professional influence in persuading a patient to accept a treatment is unethical. When things go well and the patient/family is able to respond to caring practices, the practitioner cannot attribute the good outcome solely to the efficacy of some technique they may have used.

In the recent past, nursing practice on "prespecified outcomes" identified and evaluated nursing outcomes in case management based on the premise that only technique is involved in health care, that one knows the outcomes to expect, and that all things can be "fixed." The problem is further complicated by institutional constraints to effective caregiving. Meeting and responding to the other may clash with the bureaucratic goals of care for the many in the most cost-efficient manner. For all these reasons, developing moral agency and the skills of involvement present ongoing demands for experiential learning and character development. Viewing nursing as a basic human encounter and as a practice that requires phronesis has major implications for nursing education and the moral development of practitioners.

Technical cure and restorative care must not become mutually exclusive for the nurse. One way to create more equal dialogical partners between technical health care and everyday social existence or *lifeworlds* (defined as a person's everyday way of being in a particular culture, subculture, and nexus of interpersonal relationships and social roles) is to understand medicine, nursing, and other health care practices as *practices* that encompass more than the science and technologies they use to effect cures.

Developing expert practice in local, specific settings requires experiential learning as well as communicating that experiential learning to others so that clinical knowledge is continually developed and evaluated. This experientially gained clinical knowledge is held collectively by a local group of practitioners who extend local knowledge through dialogue with larger practice communities. Communities of practitioners must find ways to make their experiential learning collective and cumulative in order for nursing practices in local settings to grow and improve. It is wasteful and harmful when experiential learning is not shared with other clinicians. Experiential learning is expensive to acquire for patients and for nurses. Improving systems and enhancing individual performance and responsibility requires a *community of local practitioners* who collectively work to improve their clinical practice.

The two dominant approaches to reducing errors in health care, a systems approach and individual practitioner learning and responsibility, both depend on local practice communities and on the larger tradition of good practice. Improving practice systems and performance of individual clinicians both depend on the socially embedded knowledge and teamwork of practitioners in local practice settings. This is another contrast between theory and practice.

Theory derives its power from the ability to be abstract and applicable over a range of particular situations. Practice is local and particular. Excellent practice

TABLE 5.1 Habits, Clinical Grasp, Inquiry, and Forethought
Habits of Thought and Action
1. Clinical grasp and clinical inquiry: Problem identification and clinical problem-solving
2. Clinical forethought: Anticipating and preventing potential problems

From Benner, P., Hooper-Kyriakidis, P., & Stannard, D. (1999). *Clinical wisdom and interventions in critical care nursing: A thinking-in-action approach.* Philadelphia: WB Saunders.

is lodged in a tradition of fostering good practice and ongoing experiential learning in local settings. The book *Clinical Wisdom and Interventions in Critical Care: A Thinking-in Action Approach* (Benner, Hooper-Kyriakidis, & Stannard, 1999) describes two major habits of thought and action involved in clinical reasoning: clinical grasp and clinical forethought. Parts of the book illustrate the ways in which these pervasive habits of thought and action "work" in relation to major goals of critical care nursing practice. However, these same habits of thought, clinical grasp, and clinical forethought can be found in all domains of nursing practice. Table 5.1 draws heavily on the original research reported in the book on clinical wisdom.

Experiential learning is risky and expensive in underdetermined, fast-paced, clinical circumstances. The clinician's goal is to be as accurate and certain as possible before acting. Habits of thought and action that foster experiential learning are not automatic. They must be cultivated through practice and reflection on practice by individuals and groups of clinicians. Attentiveness, openness to disconfirming evidence, choosing strategies for confirming hypotheses, and narrative reasoning that considers the clinician's own transitions in understanding all foster experiential learning. Careless mistakes, lack of attentiveness, and neglect are to be avoided but when they occur, the responsible clinician corrects them and refocuses on the improving practice and the system. Nurse educators in all sectors of nursing education are concerned with ways to teach ethical and clinical reasoning.

Perception or *seeing* the most salient ethical and clinical issues is the first step in responding to clinical issues. Perceptual grasp comes before *defining* the problem. Knowing ethical principles and the relevant science are of no avail if learners cannot recognize when the principles and science are at stake in actual clinical situations. Teaching and learning clinical and ethical judgment are made more complex by the rapid time demand and the necessity of moving assessments to interventions or immediate action in crisis situations.

DISTINCTIONS BETWEEN CLINICAL AND SCIENTIFIC REASONING

Clinical reasoning is distinct from scientific reasoning, even though scientific knowledge is central to good clinical reasoning. As noted earlier, clinical judgment entails reasoning about the particular across time, through transitions in the clinical condition of the patient, and through transitions in clinicians' under-standings of the patient's clinical condition. In contrast, scientific problem solving entails establishing experimental conditions where the scientist can compare experimental results at single points in time, in clearly specified contexts, in the form of absolute judgments. While scientific reasoning can be frozen in time through formal scientific study of appropriate samples, clinical reasoning cannot. Clinical reasoning relies on keeping track of narrative clinical understanding across time. Narrative reasoning across time about the particular must guide the use of critical pathways, prognostic scores, and evidence-based guidelines. Thus clinical reasoning requires an understanding of basic scientific explanations, evidence from aggregate patient populations *and* the ways in which these might be accurately interpreted in relation to particular patients. As a consequence, even expert clinicians may feel that their practice never measures up to their idealized models of scientific reasoning or making particular decisions based on aggregate data. Yet actual expert clinical reasoning is always linked with notions of good practice (ethical reasoning) and takes into account what has been learned from clinical changes in the particular patient's condition and the patient's patterns of responses to interventions over time.

In order to use good clinical reasoning, the nurse must be skillful in moral and clinical perception (Benner & Wrubel, 1982; Blum, 1994). Although conceptual knowledge is essential, it is not sufficient to ensure that the nurse will form relationships with patients that lead to salient disclosures, or that the nurse will notice and correctly identify an instance of pulmonary edema, despair, or pain when he or she sees it, even though the nurse may know conceptually what the formal characteristics of these patient conditions are in principle.

In the practice of medicine and nursing, science and technology are used to increase certainty about measurement of signs and symptoms. The practice of these objective measurements reduces errors and improves clinical reasoning. No one would recommend going back to guessing body temperatures by palpation alone. However, even the most formal measurements cannot replace the perceptual skill of the clinician in recognizing when a measurement is relevant or the meaning of a particular measurement. Also, following the course of the patient's development of signs and symptoms (the trajectory or evolution of signs and symptoms) informs the clinician's understanding of the meaning of those signs and symptoms. This may seem patently obvious to any practicing clinician, yet current strategies for applying algorithms or making particular clinical judgments based on aggregate outcomes data alone ignore the clinical know-how, relational skills, and need for clinical judgment as reasoning across time (Halpern, 2001).

Technique is defined here as prespecified outcomes that can be reduced to routine, predictable, standardized care. A more robust understanding of practice needs to be developed in an era when science and technology have become the dominant, public, legitimized discourses for modern practices.

Good nursing practice requires the development of ongoing, clinical knowledge through experiential learning. Experiential learning is not automatic. It requires openness, attentiveness, and responsible, engaged learning on the part of the practitioner. Reflection on practice and active engaged thinking are required. Here a distinction is being made between detached, disengaged reflection and engaged thinking-in-action (Benner, Hooper-Kyriakidis, & Stannard, 1999). Standing outside the situation and reflecting back on it is a powerful critical thinking strategy for improving practice, especially in situations of breakdown and error (Schon, 1987). However, being emotionally attuned to the patient/family and the demands of the situation in the immediate moment is required for well-timed expert performance.

The Dreyfus Model of Skill Acquisition (Benner, 1984, 2001; Dreyfus & Dreyfus, 1986) is based on determining the level of practice evident in particular situations. It elucidates strengths as well as problems. Situated practice capacities are described rather than traits or talents of the practitioners. At each stage of experiential learning (novice, advanced beginner, competent, proficient, expert), clinicians can perform at their best. For example, one can be the best advanced beginner possible, typically the first year of practice. However, no practitioner can be beyond experience, regardless of the level of skill acquisition in most clinical situations and despite the necessary attempts to make practice as clear and explicit as possible. If the nurse has never encountered a particular clinical situation, experiential learning is required. For example, referring to critical pathways is not the same as recognizing when and how these pathways are relevant or must be adapted to particular patients. Experiential learning that leads to individualization and clinical discernment is required to render critical pathways sensible and safe. Such individualization requires clinical discernment based on experience with past whole concrete clinical situations. This ability to make clinical comparisons between whole, concrete, clinical cases without decomposing the whole situation into its analytical components is a hallmark of expert clinical nursing practice. A renewing, coherent, recognizable identity requires that practitioners develop notions of good that are constantly being worked out and extended through experiential learning in local and larger practice communities. Practice is a way of knowing, as well as a way of being in the world (Benner, Hooper-Kyriakidis, & Stannard, 1999). A self-renewing practice directs the development, implementation, and evaluation of science and technology. Clinical judgment requires moral agency (defined as the ability to affect and influence situations), relationship, perceptual acuity, skilled know-how, and narrative reasoning across time about particular patient transitions (Benner, Hooper-Kyriakidis, & Stannard, 1999).

CLINICAL GRASP

Clinical grasp describes clinical inquiry in action. Clinical grasp includes problem identification and clinical judgment across time about the particular transitions of particular patients/families. Four aspects of clinical grasp include (1) making qualitative distinctions, (2) engaging in detective work, (3) recognizing changing relevance, and (4) developing clinical knowledge in specific patient populations.

MAKING QUALITATIVE DISTINCTIONS

Qualitative distinctions refers to those distinctions that can only be made in particular, contextual, or historical situations. In the clinical example above, the nurse was listening for qualitative changes in the breath sounds, and changes in the patient's color and also changes in the patient's mental alertness. Context and sequence of events are essential for making qualitative distinctions; therefore they require paying attention to transitions and judgment (Benner, 1994; Benner, Hooper-Kyriakidis, & Stannard, 1999). Many qualitative distinctions can only be made by observing differences through touch, sound, or sight, as in skin turgor, color, and capillary refill (Hooper, 1995).

ENGAGING IN DETECTIVE WORK, MODUS OPERANDI THINKING, AND CLINICAL REASONING

SOLVING PUZZLES

Nurse educators and regulators alike have conflated *critical thinking, scientific thinking,* and *clinical reasoning.* Clinical reasoning is always about reasoning across time about the particular through changes in the patient's concerns of condition and/or changes in the clinician's understanding of the nature of the patient's condition (Benner, Hooper-Kyriakidis, & Stannard, 1999). Nurses use scientific evidence in their clinical thinking and reasoning, but they do not "use the scientific problem-solving process," since that process is both static and linear and designed to yield convincing evidence for confirmation or disconfirmation of hypotheses according to formal criteria or operational definitions. Critical thinking is essential for examining outmoded practices, and for when there is confusion and complete puzzlement about the patient's clinical condition and the meaning of signs and symptoms. Critical thinking is a form of deconstruction and critical reflection. It critiques and judges what is wrong or puzzling, and evaluates the soundness of assumptions. But reasoning through transitions over time is required for clinical reasoning and discernment. This is a form of practical reasoning and puzzle solving that is analogous to "modus operandi" thinking (Benner, Tanner, Chesla, 2009).

Clinical situations are open ended and underdetermined. Modus operandi thinking keeps track of the particular patient, the way the illness unfolds, and the meaning of the patient's responses as they have occurred in the particular time sequence. Modus operandi thinking requires keeping track of what has been tried and what has or has not worked with the patient. In this kind of reasoning-in-transition, gains and losses in understanding that are error reducing are evaluated for their significance (Benner, Hughes, & Sutphen, 2008; Benner, 1994; Taylor, 1989, 1993). For example, an advanced practice nurse clinician reviewing a patient's x-ray considers her condition and considers the possibility of pneumothorax. He determines that a second comparative chest x-ray is needed. Later in an interview he states:

> I guess it could have been a pulmonary embolus. But I was really sort of focused on the differences and the fact that it was fairly similar in appearance, which can

happen with pulmonary emboli. The heart rhythm pattern had not changed, although it was elevated. There was some tachycardia. Uhm, but, it sort of was leading me to believe that this was more sort of a pulmonary problem as opposed to a pulmonary circulation problem, you know (Benner, Hooper-Kyriakidis, & Stannard, 1999).

The clinician is guessing that this is a problem of physical phenomenon of air moving in and out rather than obstructions to pulmonary circulation. The evidence is subtle, so the clinician stays open to disconfirmation but proceeds with attempts to obtain the chest x-ray and is prepared to recognize the sudden change in the patient's respiratory status when that occurs. Another qualitative distinction was the judgment of whether the patient's change in mental status and agitation was primarily the result of anxiety or hypoxia.

RECOGNIZING CHANGING CLINICAL RELEVANCE

Recognizing changes in clinical relevance is an experientially learned skill that enables clinicians to distinguish what is relevant in situations. The meanings of signs and symptoms are changed by sequencing and history. In the above example, the patient's mental status and color continued to deteriorate, as did the diminishment of his breath sounds. Once chest tubes were in place, a dramatic change occurred in the patient's color. Each of these changes in the patient's signs and symptoms is made by examining the transitions as they occur.

DEVELOPING CLINICAL KNOWLEDGE IN SPECIFIC PATIENT POPULATIONS

Because this clinician has had the opportunity to observe both pulmonary circulation problems and mechanical breathing problems, he is able to recognize a kind of "family resemblance" with other mechanical breathing problems (as opposed to pulmonary circulation problems) that he has noticed with other patients.

Refinement of clinical reasoning is possible when nurses have the opportunity to work with specific patient populations. The comparisons between many specific patients create a matrix of comparisons for clinicians, as well as a tacit background set of expectations that create active detective work if a patient does not meet the usual predictable transitions in recovery. What is in the background and foreground of the clinician's attention needs to shift with changes in the patient's condition. Understanding a particular patient population well can assist with recognizing these shifts.

CLINICAL FORETHOUGHT

Clinical forethought is another pervasive habit of thought and action in nursing practice evident in this narrative example (Benner, Hooper-Kyriakidis, & Stannard, 1999). Clinical forethought plays a role in clinical grasp because it structures the practical logic of clinicians. Clinical forethought refers to at least four habits of thought and action: (1) future think, (2) clinical forethought about specific patient populations, (3) anticipation of risks for particular patients, and, (4) seeing the unexpected.

FUTURE THINK

Future think is the broadest category of this logic of practice. In the example, the advanced practice nurse stated: "So I stayed in with the nurse, and we were talking and going over what the plan was and things we might be looking for in the evening." Anticipating likely immediate futures helps with making good clinical judgments and with preparing the environment so that the nurse can respond to the patient's immediate needs in a timely fashion. Essential clinical judgments and timely interventions would be impossible in rapidly changing clinical situations without lead time or anticipation, a well developed sense of salience for noticing what is most urgent in the situation, and an environment prepared for anticipated patient needs. Future think governs the style and content of the nurse's attentiveness to the patient. Whether in a fast-paced, acute care, or slower paced rehabilitation setting, thinking and acting with anticipated futures guide clinical thinking and judgment. Future think captures the way judgment is suspended in a predictive net of thoughtful planning-ahead and preparing the environment for likely eventualities.

CLINICAL FORETHOUGHT ABOUT SPECIFIC PATIENT POPULATIONS

This habit of thought and action is so second nature to the experienced nurse that he or she may neglect to tell the newcomer, the "obvious." Clinical forethought involves much local, specific knowledge, such as who is a good resource and how to marshal support services and equipment for particular patients. The staff nurse used good judgment in calling the advanced practice nurse to assist in solving the puzzle when she was unable to convince the less clinically experienced junior resident. The advanced practice nurse made use of all available physicians in the area. Part of what made a timely response possible was the actual planning of a situation that might change rapidly.

Examples of preparing for specific patient populations abound in all settings. Examples including anticipating the need for a pacemaker during surgery and having the equipment assembled ready for use saves essential time, or forecasting an accident victim's potential injuries when intubation might be needed for the accident victim.

ANTICIPATION OF RISKS FOR PARTICULAR PATIENTS

This narrative example is shaped by the foreboding sense of an impending crisis for this particular patient. A staff nurse uses her sense of nervousness or uneasiness about the changes in a patient's breathing to initiate her problem search. This aspect of clinical forethought is central to knowing the particular patient, family, or community. Nurses situate the patient's problems almost like a topography of possibilities. This vital clinical knowledge needs to be communicated to other caregivers and across care borders.

Clinical teaching could be improved by enriching curricula with narratives from actual practice and by helping students recognize commonly occurring clinical situations. For example, if a patient is hemodynamically unstable, then managing life-sustaining physiologic functions will be a main orienting goal. If a patient is agitated and uncomfortable, then attending to comfort needs in relation to hemodynamics will be a priority (Benner, Hooper-Kyriakidis, & Stannard, 1999). Providing comfort measures emerges as a central background practice for making clinical judgments, and contains within it much judgment and experiential learning. When clinical teaching is too removed from typical contingencies and strong clinical situations in practice, students will lack practice in active thinking-in-action in ambiguous clinical situations. With the rapid advance of knowledge and technology, students need to be good clinical learners and clinical knowledge developers. One way nurse educators can enhance clinical inquiry is by increasing experiential learning in the curriculum.

Experiential learning requires open learning climates where students can discuss and examine transitions in understanding including their false starts or their misconceptions in actual clinical situations. Focusing *only* on performance and on "being correct" and not on learning from breakdown or error dampens students' curiosity and courage to learn experientially.

One's *sense* of moral agency, as well as *actual* moral agency, in particular situations changes with level of skill acquisition (Benner, Hooper-Kyriakidis, & Stannard 1999; Benner, 2005). Furthermore, experiential learning is facilitated or hampered by learning skills of involvement with patients/families and engagement with clinical problems at hand. Those nurses who do not go on to become expert clinicians have some learning difficulty associated with skills of involvement, and consequently with making clinical judgments, particularly making qualitative distinctions (Benner, Hooper-Kyriakidis, & Stannard, 1999; Benner, Tanner, & Chesla, 1996). Experienced, nonexpert nurses see clinical problem solving as a simple weighing of facts or rational calculation. They do not experience their own agency in making clinical judgments. They fail to see qualitative distinctions linked to the patient's well being.

SEEING THE UNEXPECTED

One of the keys to becoming an expert practitioner lies in the ways in which the practitioner holds past experiential learning and background habitual skills and practices. If nothing is considered routine, as a habitual response pattern, then practitioners cannot function in emergencies attending to the unexpected. However, if expectations are held rigidly, then subtle changes from the usual will be missed and habitual and rote responses will rule. The clinician must be flexible in shifting between what is in the background and the foreground. This is accomplished by staying curious and open. The clinical "certainty" associated with perceptual grasp is distinct from the kind of "certainty" achievable in scientific experiments and through measurements. It is similar to "face recognition" or recognition of "family resemblances." It is subject to faulty memory, false associative memories, and mistaken identities; therefore such perceptual grasp is the beginning of curiosity and inquiry and not the end (Benner, Hooper-Kyriakidis, & Stannard, 1999; Benner, Chesla, & Tanner, 2009).

In rapidly moving clinical situations, perceptual grasp is the starting point for clarification, confirmation, and action. The relationship between the foreground and the background of attention needs to be fluid so that missed expectations allow the nurse to *see* the unexpected. For example, when the background rhythm of a cardiac monitor changes, the nurse notices, and what had been background tacit awareness becomes the foreground of attention. A hallmark of expertise is the ability to notice the unexpected (Benner, Hooper-Kyriakidis, & Stannard, 1999). Background expectations of usual patient trajectories form with experience. These background experiences form tacit expectations that enable the nurse to notice subtle failed expectations and pay attention to early signs of unexpected changes in the patient's condition. Clinical expectations gained from caring for similar patient populations form a tacit *clinical forethought* that enables the experienced clinician to notice missed expectations. Alterations from implicit or explicit expectations set the stage for experiential learning depending on the openness of the learner.

DIAGNOSTIC DISCERNMENT, MORAL AGENCY, AND ADVOCACY

Moral agency relies on more than will and intent (Sherman, 1997). The Kantian tradition is insufficient for practice disciplines in that it focuses primarily on will and intent, and overlooks moral agency as the ability to respond emotionally and act in relation to notions of "good" (Kant, 1785). Aristotle, in 322 B.C., noted that carrying out and acting on moral principles requires the development of character and skill in a social context. For example, given the same moral intentions, the experienced expert nurse will be able to exercise moral agency in a complex situation because of perceptual acuity, skilled know-how, and social competence gained in a particular social setting. However, the beginning nurse may be too caught up with the tasks at hand, lack adequate perceptual acuity to recognize the moral infraction, or lack the social understanding and influence to make the appropriate corrective response to the situation.

Intelligent and timely advocacy requires critical thinking that enables the nurse to evaluate the level and adequacy of medical treatment and nursing care for the patient. As noted, this requires sufficient time for the nurse to meet and attend to the patient. For example, if a patient misunderstands the implications of a medical treatment or nursing intervention, then the nurse must assist the patient in clarifying the implications, consequences, and potential side effects. Advocacy may be involved in helping a patient understand the need for an unpleasant medical procedure, such as the insertion of a nasogastric tube and subsequent suctioning, when the patient is suffering from vomiting and distention due to a gastrointestinal blockage.

Advocacy is more than ensuring the "consumer's preferences." It requires understanding the patient's plight, understanding the concerns in relation to the potential benefits of medical treatments and nursing interventions, and working with the patient to confront difficult decisions. Advocacy must place the patient's autonomy and choices first. But the expectation goes further to help patients better understand and assess the implications of their decision.

DIAGNOSTIC DISCERNMENT AND THE ENVIRONMENT OF CARE

Many environmental factors exist in health care systems that influence the decisions that nurses make while providing nursing care. In the ideal workplace, the nurse is able to make sound, professional, and humane nursing decisions based on extensive knowledge, clinical skills, competency, and time to make decisions. A culture of safety informs the work environment so that a context exists without serious organizational structure or process impediments and in which a nurse can exercise sound clinical judgment and implement decision-making skills. Sound practice requires a work environment that reinforces and sustains the notions of good practice internal to the practice.

Unfortunately, many impediments within a health care setting do exist. These may hinder a nurse's ability to make the best clinical decision and will often force a choice between implementing the best course of action for the patient or modifying best care standards based on poor policies or inadequate resources within the workplace.

DIAGNOSTIC DISCERNMENT AND THE MARKETPLACE

Assuring adequate nurse staffing has been affected by significant cost-cutting initiatives throughout the health care system. Unfortunately, the evidence or lack of evidence for such decisions has often resulted in negative patient outcomes, nurse frustration, and increased long-term costs. Examples of several of the factors impacting nurse staffing include:

1. The worsening nursing shortage coupled with the aging of the nurse workforce.
2. An aging population that is associated with increased demand for health care.
3. Increased expectations for health care organizations to operate within a business model framework (Aiken, Sochalski, & Anderson, 1996).
4. Decreased reimbursement for health care services.
5. Increased competition for staff.
6. A health care system increasingly driven by free market competition coupled with escalating costs of health care services.
7. Use of efficiency-driven institutional policies often at odds with effective, safe health care delivery practices.
8. Expectations for safe staffing ratios, job descriptions, philosophy of care, and allocation of resources to support profit making at the expense of patient care outcomes.
9. Expectations for the licensed nurse to "delegate" and/or assume additional roles in a climate that does not reflect the standard of nursing practice that may be optimal for the patient for which unlicensed personnel have been inadequately prepared (Aiken et al., 2001).

10. Efforts to reduce costs by decreasing the number of registered nurses and increasing the number of unlicensed nursing assistants and support caregivers.
11. An acute shortage of nursing faculty so that it is impossible to increase the capacities of nursing schools to accommodate the number of new entrants into the profession required (Buerhaus, Staiger, & Auerbach, 2000).
12. Consumer awareness and demand driving changes in the way health care is delivered. An increasing number of patients and families are requesting home care rather than traditional hospitalization and/or long-term care and are demanding to play an active role in the care they receive.
13. The proliferation of clinical monitoring technology available for health care services. The use of technology requires increasingly greater registered nurse time and attention to individual patients, many of whom are now placed in ICUs and step-down units for intensive, highly technical care. Clinical monitoring technology has also influenced the way health care is delivered. A larger percentage of critically ill patients survive and have shorter inpatient stays in the acute care hospital setting but still require skilled nursing care outside of acute care hospitals. This has resulted in an upward shift in the acuity of patients in nursing homes, assisted living/residential care facilities, and home care. Many times these facilities are licensed by the state and certified through Medicare. These regulations often do not reflect the acuity of their current patient population.
14. Advances in documentation technology that have changed the way nurses communicate. Nurses now often communicate by computer with nursing colleagues, physicians, pharmacists, and those to whom they delegate, resulting in an electronic format and approach to medical records. Currently this change to computerized medical records is promising though uneven in different health care actions. For example, an electronic record may improve the accuracy of documentation of vital signs, decreasing the error rate to 5% (Gearing et al., 2006). A study by Singh, Servoss, Kalsman, Fox, & Singh (2004) demonstrated a decreased sense of threat for patient safety in nurse-physician and physician-chart interactions, but an increased risk in physician-patient assessment and nurse-chart interactions. The authors conclude that through electronic records the visibility and awareness of other problem areas may increase, and indeed electronic records may create *new* problems that do not show up until the system is in place and tested over time.

When working environments are less than optimal, the infrastructure for safe and effective diagnostic discernment is most likely absent, and negative patient outcomes may result. Work environment design and efficiency models have become major driving factors of patient care outcomes. In this regard, nurses are not able to overcome all the impediments to providing safe levels of monitoring and surveillance. Complaints filed with state boards of nursing frequently reflect the unstable and unsafe working environments in the health care system.

CHALLENGES IN DEVELOPING SKILLS IN DIAGNOSTIC DISCERNMENT

Nurses enter the workforce after they complete their undergraduate work. They believe that they have learned the basic elements of the profession and that they will be able to provide safe and competent nursing care in their chosen health care setting. This belief is supported by the *Report of Findings From the Practice and Professional Issues Survey 2002* (NCSBN, 2003) in which newly licensed and practicing nurses reported feeling competent to perform basic nursing procedures, such as "administer medications by common routes" and to "provide direct care to two or more clients." However, the practices these respondents reported about which they did not feel competent included "provide direct care to six or more clients"; communication and management skills required to "supervise care provided by others"; and "know when and how to call a client's physician." If the educational institution or the employer does not provide this school-to-work and day-to-day practice transition skills, the care delivered may be compromised during the initial period of learning.

Another factor that impacts acceptable practice is the gap between the regulatory board's defined scope of practice for the licensed nurse and state and federal regulations that define the minimum licensure and certification requirements of health care agencies. These gaps suggest that coordination and institutional design are not congruent with the newly graduated nurse's actual capacities to provide safe nursing care throughout the full range of current health care environments. Specifically, these may include the gaps between the licensed nurse's confidence in his/her ability to practice safely, the errors that occur in heath care environments new to the nurse, and the policies of the various health care agencies in which nurses practice. These gaps call for improved educational programs and better transition from school to work in practice settings. *The Carnegie National Nursing Education Study,* based on Sullivan's work, has identified three apprenticeships as essential to professional education (Benner, Sutphen, Leonard, & Day., in press; Sullivan, 2005). To capture the full range of crucial dimensions in professional education, the organizations developed the idea of a threefold apprenticeship: (1) intellectual training to learn the academic knowledge base and the capacity to think in ways important to the profession, (2) a skill-based apprenticeship of practice (and clinical judgment), and (3) an apprenticeship to the ethical standards, social roles, and responsibilities of the profession through which the novice is introduced to the meaning of an integrated practice of all dimensions of the profession grounded in the profession's fundamental purposes. The creators of this initiative noted: "This framework has allowed us to describe tensions and shortfalls as well as strengths of widespread teaching practices, especially at articulation points among these dimensions of professional training" (Benner et al., in press, p. 7).

Aristotle linked experiential learning to the development of character and moral sensitivities of a person learning a practice (Dunne, 1997). In the

Carnegie studies of professional education, the development of moral character is called "formation" by the clergy. Good teaching practices seek to integrate all three apprenticeships so that students will learn how to intertwine these three essential apprenticeships in their practice. No doubt rational calculations available to *techne*—population trends and statistics, and algorithms created as decision support structures—can improve accuracy when used as a stance of inquiry in making clinical judgments about particular patients. Ultimately, however, the skills of *phronesis* will be required for nursing, medicine, or any helping professional (Dunne, 1997). Specifically, these refer to clinical reasoning that reasons across time, taking into account the transitions of the particular patient/family/ community and transitions in the clinician's understanding of the clinical situation. As noted in Chapter 4, good clinical judgment requires adequate institutional design, time, and support, nurse monitoring, and attentiveness to allow for nurses to adequately monitor and spend time with patients. Good clinical reasoning is facilitated when the nurse knows the patient and is able to pay attention to changes in the patient over time. Delegated monitoring and vital sign assessments must be communicated clearly. Good clinical reasoning is also facilitated when the nurse has in-depth knowledge of the particular patient population in question. Understanding usual patient recovery trajectories in a patient population helps nurses recognize deviations from the usual recovery trajectory.

Clinical reasoning is affected by the context of care. If the nurse is not familiar with a patient population, a resource nurse should be made available for consultation and cross-checking of the patient. When a patient crisis drains the staff resources to attend to all patients on the unit, the supervisory staff must have a plan in place to provide additional staff support during these times of high demands. It is crucial to sort out causes of poor clinical judgments, breakdowns in monitoring and attentiveness, inadequate patient history or information, lack of knowledge about the relevant clinical signs, and the symptoms to be observed.

HISTORICAL CASE STUDY #1: When Nursing Care and More Complex and Adequate Training and Supervision Are Absent

ENVIRONMENT AND HISTORY

This case took place in a small rural community of 8000 people. Mr. Kenny Salamino was a developmentally and physically disabled 32-year-old man. He had lived most of his life in a group home with seven other residents and was cared for by a staff of two unlicensed assistive personnel (UAP) 24 hours a day.

Ms. Marsha Mitchell, a licensed practical nurse whose title was "Medical Director," had worked at the group home Monday through Friday, 8 AM to 5 PM, for 7 years. Ms. Rose Sinclair, a registered nurse, served as "Consultant." Nurse Sinclair was employed to "be a resource" and provide a course entitled "Assistance With Medications Course for Unlicensed Assistive Personnel." The owner of the facility, Mr. Brian Adams, did not live at or maintain an office at the facility. He hired the staff and expected the registered nurse and the licensed practical nurse to manage the resident care.

The state board of nursing in which the facility was located received a complaint from the Department of Health and Welfare. Mr. Salamino had died after admission to the hospital, and the state's surveyors from the Bureau of Facility Standards had investigated the circumstances of his death. Over a period of 6 months, Mr. Salamino had lost 40 pounds during which time the nurses had not assessed his health care needs or provided for adequate medical or nursing interventions. The bureau's investigation determined that the events that led to Mr. Salamino's death were due to lack of fiduciary responsibility of Practical Nurse Mitchell and Nurse Sinclair who, the report asserted, should be held accountable for Mr. Salamino's death.

THE NURSES' STORY

I have been a registered nurse for 10 years. I worked full time in a small hospital in a nearby town for 9 years as the supervising registered nurse. When I decided to work part-time, I chose to drop back and work in a less restricted environment than the hospital. The administrator of the group home hired me as the "Registered Nurse Consultant," and my responsibilities included teaching to new unlicensed assistive personnel a course entitled "Assistance With Medications Course" and providing to the licensed practical nurse 24/7 support face to face or by cellular phone.

My contract specified that I was to be paid for 24 hours of work every 3 months. I did not receive an orientation to residential care/group home, federal, and/or state regulations.

The first indication I had that Mr. Salamino was having a problem was when Practical Nurse Mitchell called me and said that Mr. Salamino had just returned from the hospital with a new jejunostomy tube (J-tube). She said that she thought Mr. Salamino should have been discharged to a skilled nursing facility, but his physician, Dr. Fred Stark, sent him back to the group home because he thought Mr. Salamino would receive better care there. Dr. Stark worked with Practical Nurse Mitchell and the patients in the group home. They knew and loved Mr. Salamino.

I asked Practical Nurse Mitchell if she could handle the J-tube. She said she could, and thus I did not go to the group home to assess Mr. Salamino or to confirm Practical Nurse Mitchell's competency. I did not believe this was part of my job.

THE LICENSED PRACTICAL NURSE'S PERSPECTIVE

I could tell Mr. Salamino was losing weight over several months. I didn't become concerned at first because he continued to feed himself and didn't appear to be hungry. After several months, I called his doctor and he told me to bring Mr. Salamino in for a checkup. Dr. Stark was concerned about Mr. Salamino's weight loss and ran some tests. He had something wrong with his digestive tract and wasn't absorbing his food.

Dr. Stark arranged for a consult with a surgeon and that's when they decided to insert a stomach tube. Mr. Salamino was in the hospital for 2 days and was then transferred back to the group home. He was able to swallow and drink liquids. He didn't have a pump for his feedings when he arrived, so I called and ordered the pump and the liquid feeding solution that Dr. Stark had ordered. I didn't worry too much about the fact it took 4 days to start the feedings because Mr. Salamino continued to drink liquids.

When the pump and feeding solution arrived, I hooked it up but couldn't get the pump to run. I called Dr. Stark who arranged for me to take Mr. Salamino to the emergency room and meet the surgeon, Dr. Hari Harimoto. Dr. Harimoto discovered that something was wrong at the insertion site on his stomach. He repaired the insertion site and sent Mr. Salamino back to the group home. The aides and I gave Mr. Salamino his feedings as Dr. Harimoto ordered, but he developed a fever, was readmitted to the hospital about 2 weeks later, and died the same day.

When I looked back on the events that took place, I felt I was left to do everything myself. I wished Nurse Sinclair would have been more involved in what was going on, but she said she was not hired to see the residents. I know we gave Mr. Salamino better care than he would have gotten at the nursing home. They have too many patients and not enough nurses.

THE ADMINISTRATOR'S PERSPECTIVE

I have owned this facility for 15 years and never had a problem until this happened. Practical Nurse Mitchell is a good licensed practical nurse and handles things perfectly fine. I don't see any reason to have to pay a registered nurse to do what Practical Nurse Mitchell, a licensed practical nurse, can do on her own. I didn't see any reason to orient the registered nurse or licensed practical nurse to residential care/group home regulations. They are supposed to take care of the residents.

CASE ANALYSIS

This case demonstrates the classic example of the common expectation that residential/group home care does not require the level of nursing skill and attentiveness that is required in a hospital or skilled nursing facility. This expectation persists despite the fact that residents change in their care needs, and the home may not be able to keep up with the technical care demands of these changes. This owner-established care supervision plan was inadequate given the nature of the changes in the care the patient required. Several actions were inadequate in this series of events regarding the decisions that affected the patient's well-being. The practice breakdown elements included the following:

1. The administrator of the group home did not provide orientation for the registered nurse immediately after her arrival. Consequently she was unaware that the State Regulations for Residential Care Facilities required that a registered nurse assesses patients on a regular basis to identify any health care needs that may be developing and to refer the patient for medical care as

needed. It was only when the patient died that the state surveyed the facility and discovered the lack of supervision of a registered nurse.

2. The administrator failed to provide adequate resources for the registered nurse and licensed practical nurse in their respective roles. The registered nurse was only paid for 24 hours of work in a 3-month period. She understood that her role was to provide the course "Assistance With Medications Course" for newly hired unlicensed assistive personnel, but this responsibility alone took more than the 24 hours for which she was paid. She did not understand that she was in a role that required her participation and direction for the care of the patients in the facility. She did not recognize her role as a "registered nurse consultant" to be "anything more than a registered nurse available on the cellular phone 24 hours per day." She was not expected by administration to assume responsibility for assessment of the patients and/or to collaborate with the licensed practical nurse and physician.

3. Practical Nurse Mitchell had the title "Medical Director," which led her to believe that she was to make all decisions related to patient care. The licensed practical nurse was reluctant to call the registered nurse when she had concerns. She did contact the physician, but she did not identify the patient's health issues until the patient required hospitalization. The health care system in which the licensed practical nurse and registered nurse practiced did not design, mandate, or pay for the support and guidance that a registered nurse should have provided.

4. After the first hospitalization, the patient's physician discharged his patient to the group home. The physician believed that the patient would receive better care in his "home," where the staff was familiar with him, rather than refer him to a skilled nursing facility that could provide the skilled care he required. However, this group home was not adequately prepared to provide the skilled nursing care he needed.

The licensed practical nurse did not doubt her ability to administer medications by common routes and to provide care to two or more patients. But the evidence in this case did not address the competencies required for tube feeding and recognizing malnutrition. Further, the licensed practical nurse was slow to contact the physician regarding the patient's emerging physical changes, which could have been due to either a reluctance to call the physician and/or her lack of assessment or awareness of the dangerous level of weight loss and malnourishment.

Both nurses in this case were not aware that their individual levels of nursing education applied in this setting. The descriptions of their positions defined the relationship between the registered nurse and the licensed practical nurse. The licensed practical nurse was "in charge," and the registered nurse was hired as a figurehead to meet the administrator's interpretation of the requirements for licensure of a group facility. These institutional policies established the scenario that eventually resulted in a patient's death. The licensed practical nurse assumed responsibility for all patient care but did not have the skills or support from the registered nurse to identify the patient's initial life-threatening weight loss, and later the need for timely initiation of his tube feedings. She continued to deal with the situation alone rather than contact and consult with the registered nurse and physician to determine the actions needed. Because the registered nurse had never worked in residential care before and was unaware of the federal and state requirements for residential care, she assumed that the duties as written in her position description were appropriate. Based on these duties, she did not assume a supervisory or active collaborative role to support the licensed practical nurse. The registered nurse and the licensed practical nurse did not question the scope of the duties in descriptions of their respective positions, nor did they look to the Nurse Practice Act and Administrative Rules to identify the roles their state board required for each respective nursing license or question their "positions" at the time they were hired. The registered nurse was content to have minimal collaborative responsibility and limited hours. The licensed practical nurse did not recognize that she lacked sufficient knowledge and training to provide the more skilled nursing care involved in tube feeding a patient through a jejunostomy. Further, the licensed practical nurse was flattered by her title and did not question the fact that she was not appropriately educated and competent to manage and provide adequate nursing care without support.

HISTORICAL CASE STUDY #2: When Short Staffing Hinders Good Clinical Reasoning

ENVIRONMENT AND HISTORY

This case took place in a local hospital of a community of 50,000 people. Mr. Jim Luke, a registered nurse assigned to the ICU/CCU during the night shift, had been working part-time in this unit for about 2 years and had been licensed for 8 years. His previous experience included medical-surgical nursing and working in a cardiac catheterization lab. Nurse Luke said he had not received any orientation or additional training when he was transferred to the ICU/CCU.

The board of nursing received a complaint from the hospital after a patient, Mr. John Clark, had died. The allegations were that Nurse Luke had oversedated Mr. Clark, had used chemical restraints to control Mr. Clark's behavior, and that Nurse Luke's actions had contributed to Mr. Clark's death.

THE NURSE'S STORY

I was the registered nurse who admitted the patient, Mr. John Clark, to the ICU/CCU from the medical-surgical floor the previous night. Mr. Clark was a 73-year-old man with multiple diagnoses including acute pancreatitis, acute respiratory failure, pneumonia, chronic airway obstruction, atrial fibrillation, congestive heart failure, and hypertension. Mr. Clark was confused and complained of pain. He was quite restless and frequently tried to get out of bed. He was started on BiPAP when admitted to the ICU/CCU. His wife had been sitting with him during the nights he was in the medical-surgical unit, and she also sat with him during the night he was admitted to the ICU/CCU.

When I arrived the next night for my shift I was given the report and told there were five patients in the ICU/CCU, including Mr. Clark and four patients who had been transferred from the medical-surgical unit just prior to the shift change. The additional patients included an 85-year-old female with neutropenia who required isolation, a 41-year-old female with a kidney stone, a 22-month-old female with respiratory syncytial virus who required isolation, and an 86-year-old female with congestive heart failure.

According to our infection control policy, the patient with neutropenia and the patient with a virus could not be assigned to the same nurse. One other registered nurse was also assigned to the unit. We did not have a unit clerk or an aide assigned to the unit. I objected and said we would need additional help. The nursing supervisor told me that the patients were not as acutely ill as the usual ICU/CCU patients and, therefore, we did not need additional staffing. I pointed out that two of the patients required isolation procedures and this not only took extra time for the nurses to gown and mask but also no one was available to watch the other patients when the nurses were in the rooms with the door closed with the isolation patients. I was told that this was not an issue and that the staffing was adequate. I asked if there was another registered nurse on call but was told by the nurse supervisor that I did not have authorization to call her in for assistance. I again requested additional help because the admissions for the additional patients were not completed. This would take additional time. Again, the request was denied.

When I began the shift, Ms. Clark was sitting with her husband who was restless and agitated. Mr. Clark said he wanted to go to another hospital and was trying to get out of bed. His wife was able to calm him, but she had been sitting with him every night for over a week and was very tired. I completed my assessments for the shift, and a short time later another patient was transferred to the ICU/CCU from the emergency room, a 17-year-old patient who had overdosed.

I checked on Mr. Clark, who was still agitated, and his wife told me she needed some rest. I arranged for her to sleep in the lounge. Mr. Clark had physician orders in his chart for morphine sulfate IV 2 mg prn q2h, Benadryl 50 mg IV prn sleep HS, Inapsine 2.5 mg IV prn nausea/vomiting q6h, Ativan 1-2 mg IV prn q4h severe agitation, and Phenergan 12.5 mg IV prn nausea/vomiting q1h.

Mr. Clark was complaining of back pain, and I administered morphine sulfate IM 2 mg at 11:00 PM. Mr. Clark calmed down and appeared to be sleeping 15 minutes later.

Again, I requested an additional registered nurse, but this was refused again. The shift continued to be very busy, and at 1:30 AM I checked on Mr. Clark and found him standing beside the bed and talking about leaving the hospital. I assisted him to bed and gave him the IV Benadryl and Inapsine. Thirty minutes later, Mr. Clark was still agitated. I administered Ativan and morphine, and Mr. Clark settled down and fell asleep.

At 3:00 AM I assessed Mr. Clark, and he was sleeping with minimal respiratory effort and breath sounds were diminished with upper quadrant wheezes.

This was not a change from previous assessments. Mr. Clark continued to rest quietly throughout the shift. Nurses notes indicated: "minimal respiratory effort, shallow respirations, moves little air." I reported off to the day shift nurse and included the medication I had administered to Mr. Clark in my report.

When the day shift nurse entered Mr. Clark's room to do her assessment, she found him in sinus tachycardia with diminished breath sounds and having brief periods of apnea. He was lethargic and only withdrew from pain. The physician was called in, and Mr. Clark was placed on a ventilator. Mr. Clark's condition continued to decline and he died one week later due to complications of pancreatitis, systemic inflammatory response syndrome, respiratory failure, progressive renal insufficiency, and sepsis.

CASE ANALYSIS

Hamric, in *Reflections on Being in the Middle* (2001), states that "nurses are expected to be trustworthy team members in hierarchical top-down systems while at the same time working from the base up so as to meet patient and family needs" (p. 254). In this case, the registered nurse was caught between a nonresponsive hospital hierarchy and the dilemma of choosing the most appropriate means to protect the patient from harm.

The registered nurse recognized immediately the potential issues that could possibly arise from the staffing that was scheduled for his shift. He requested additional nursing and support staff, and the supervising/managerial personnel refused to listen to his concerns and did not accept his logic for making the request. He was forced to acquiesce to his superiors' decisions and felt he should not continue to pursue his request for additional staff.

At the beginning of the shift, the patient's wife was with him and able to calm and protect him from his confused and agitated mental state. However, she was unable to continue to be by her husband's side throughout the shift. When she left to sleep in another room, the patient was left alone without her support. The registered nurse recognized that the patient would need additional surveillance and assessed him to determine his needs. Because the patient exhibited signs of pain, the registered nurse medicated him for pain and it did calm the patient for a period of time. The admission of a new patient to the floor diverted more attention from the case study patient. Finally, in a misguided but understandable decision, the registered nurse chose to give the patient additional medication to calm him. When this did not work, he made the same decision again and administered additional medication before the effects of the previous medications were apparent. This resulted in oversedation of the patient.

Both the patient and the registered nurse paid the price for a system that did not allow for flexible decision making in order to best protect the patient from harm. Nurse Luke did not adequately recognize the significance of the patient's decreased respiratory efforts that resulted from overmedication. An additional nurse may have prevented this scenario from ending as it did. It is probable that an unlicensed individual assigned to be with Mr. Clark could have prevented this outcome had nonchemical means been provided to comfort and reassure the patient.

Nurse Luke was reported to the board of nursing for being grossly negligent and reckless in performing nursing functions and for endangering a patient. The hospital employee who reported the nurse to the board was responsible for protecting the hospital's State Licensure and Medicare Certification status in the shadow of an allegation that one of their nurse employees had used chemical restraints to subdue a patient. An experienced nurse, committed to his practice and attempting to protect a patient, made a quick, inappropriate clinical judgment in the context of work overload and a poor staffing mix that could have been prevented had the system provided additional resources.

References

Aiken, L. H., Clarke, S. P., Sloane, D. M., Sochalski, J. A., Busse, R., Clarke, H., et al. (2001). Nurses' reports on hospital care in five countries. *Health Affairs, 20*(3), 43-53.

Aiken, L. H., Sochalski, J., & Anderson, G. F. (1996). Downsizing the hospital nursing workforce. *Health Affairs, 15*(4), 88-92.

Aristotle. (1985). *Nicomachean ethics* (T. Irwin, Trans.) Indianapolis: Hackett Publishing Co. (Original work published 322 B.C.)

Benner, P., Hughes, R. G., & Sutphen, M. (2008). Clinical reasoning, decision making, and action: thinking critically and clinically. In R. G. Hughes (Ed.), *Patient safety and quality: An evidence-based handbook for nurses*. Rockville, MD: AHRQ. Available online at *http://www.ahrq.gov/qual/nurseshdbk/*. Accessed October 2, 2008.

Benner, P. (1984, 2001). *From novice to expert: Excellence and power in clinical nursing practice*. First edition and Commemorative Edition. Upper Saddle River, NJ: Prentice-Hall.

Benner, P. (1994). The role of articulation in understanding practice and experience as sources of knowledge. In J. Tully & D. M. Weinstock (Eds.), *Philosophy in a time of pluralism: Perspectives on the philosophy of Charles Taylor* (pp. 136-155). Cambridge: Cambridge University Press.

Benner, P., Hooper-Kyriakidis, P., & Stannard, D. (1999). *Clinical wisdom and interventions in critical care: A thinking-in-action approach*. Philadelphia: W.B. Saunders.

Benner, P., Sutphen, M., Leonard-Kahn, V., & Day, L. (In press). *Educating nurses: A call for radical transformation*. Carnegie Foundation for Advancement of Teaching. San Francisco: Jossey-Bass.

Benner, P., Tanner, C., & Chesla, C. (2009). *Expertise in nursing practice: Caring, clinical judgment and ethics*. New York: Springer.

Benner, P., & Wrubel, J. (1982). Skilled clinical knowledge: The value of perceptual awareness. *Nurse Educator, 7*(3), 11-17.

Blum, L. (1994). *Moral perception and particularity*. Cambridge: Cambridge University Press.

Buerhaus, P. I., Staiger, D. O., & Auerbach, D. I. (2000). Implications of an aging registered nurse workforce. *Journal of the American Medical Association, 283*(22), 2948-2954.

Dreyfus, H. L. (1992). *What computers still can't do: A critique of artificial reason.* Cambridge: Massachusetts Institute of Technology Press.

Dreyfus, H. L., & Dreyfus, S. E. (1986). *Mind over machine: The power of human intuition and expertise in the era of the computer.* New York: Free Press.

Dreyfus, H. L., Dreyfus, S. E., & Benner, P. (1996). Implications of the phenomenology of expertise for teaching and learning everyday skillful ethical comportment. In P. Benner, C. A. Tanner, & C. A. Chesla (Eds.), *Expertise in nursing practice, caring, clinical judgment and ethics* (pp. 258-279). New York: Springer.

Gearing, P., Olney, C. M., Davis, K., Lozano, D., Smith, L. B., & Friedman, B. (2006). Enhancing patient safety through electronic medical record documentation of vital signs. *Journal of Healthcare Information Management, 20*(4), 40-45.

Guignon, C. B. (1983). *Heidegger and the problem of knowledge.* Indianapolis: Hackett.

Halpern, J. (2001). *From detached concern to empathy: Humanizing medical care.* Oxford: Oxford University Press.

Hamric, A. B. (2001). Reflections on being in the middle. *Nursing Outlook, 49*(6), 254-257.

Hooper, P. (1995). *Expert titration of multiple vasoactive drugs in post-cardiac surgical patients: An interpretive study of clinical judgment and perceptual acuity.* Doctoral Dissertation, San Francisco: University of California, San Francisco School of Nursing.

Kant, I. (1785). *Critique of pure reason* (N.K. Smith, Trans., 1929). London: Macmillan.

National Council of State Boards of Nursing (NCSBN). (2003). *Report of Findings from the Practice and Professional Issues Survey, Spring 2002.* Chicago: NCSBN.

Rubin, J. (1996). Impediments to the development of clinical knowledge and ethical judgment in critical care nursing. In P. Benner, C. A. Tanner, & C. A. Chesla (Eds.), *Expertise in nursing practice, caring, clinical judgment and ethics* (pp. 269-311). New York: Springer.

Schon, D. (1987). *Educating the reflective practitioner.* San Francisco: Jossey-Bass.

Sherman, N. (1997). *Making a necessity of virtue: Aristotle and Kant on virtue.* Cambridge: Cambridge University Press.

Singh, R., Servoss, T., Kalsman, M., Fox, C., & Singh, G. (2004). Estimating impacts on safety caused by the introduction of electronic medical records in primary care. *Informatics in Primary Care, 12*(4), 235-242.

Sullivan, W. M. (2005). *Work and integrity: The crisis and promise of professionalism in America.* San Francisco: Jossey-Bass.

Taylor, C. (1989). *Sources of the self.* Cambridge, MA: Harvard University Press.

Taylor, C. (1993). Explanation and practical reason. In M. Nussbaum & A. Sen. (Eds.), *The quality of life* (pp. 208-231). Oxford: Clarendon Press.

Vetleson, A. J. (1994). *Perception, empathy, and judgment: An inquiry into the preconditions of moral performance.* University Park, PA: Pennsylvania State University Press.

6

Practice Breakdown: Prevention

Karen Bowen ◆ *Karla Bitz* ◆ *Patricia Benner*

Chapter Outline

In nursing practice, *prevention* is not always as recognizable. However *the lack of prevention* is identified by poor outcomes due to the complications of immobility and the common risks of hospitalization. Almost every aspect of nursing care involves prevention. Prevention occurs when the nurse follows usual and customary measures to prevent risks, hazards, or complications due to illness or hospitalization (NCSBN, 2006).

In the past, health care providers have not attended to prevention (Sprenger, 2001), especially within the context of patient safety. Prevention, however, is central to quality improvement. In patient safety literature the focus has been on establishing error, with emphasis on the individual and the events immediately surrounding an incident. Despite the fact that prevention constitutes such an integral component of nursing practice and quality of care, it is difficult to describe. The *lack of prevention* is more definable, visible, and measurable by the complications left behind (e.g., ventilator-acquired pneumonia, decubitus ulcers, muscle contractures, and so on).

It is not possible to identify the incidence of medical errors that are prevented each year. Active ongoing preventive measures are required for patient safety and the avoidance of adverse events and/or complications (Liolios, 2003).

Systems solutions that incorporate human factor considerations will both minimize the likelihood of error occurrence and maximize the likelihood of rapid error containment so that patient harm is averted when an error occurs (Kizer, 2001). According to Dr. James Bagian, director of the Veterans Administration National Center for Patient Safety, health care facilities and individuals need to refocus their commitment to patient safety (Tokarski, 2001), and we would add quality improvement. Specifically, a system of checks and balances must be implemented within health care organizations in order to promote safety. The blame and shame culture, lack of user-friendly error-reporting mechanisms, fear of loss of employment, and fear of litigation need to be eliminated in order for individuals to be willing to come forward and report errors for the sake of instituting redesign and the implementation of preventive measures (Kizer, 2001; Marx, 2001). For example, Bagian suggests that instead of asking, "Whose fault is this?" after the 1986 Challenger space shuttle explosion, the questions became "What happened?" and "Why?" (Tokarski, 2001).

REPORTING TO LEARN AND REDESIGN THE SYSTEM

If the hospital culture has not progressed to a "just culture" focused on practice improvement and prevention, then incident reports are likely to be perceived as punitive in the work environment. Also, if nothing changes as a result of reporting the error or a near miss, it may seem to the worker that it is a waste of time to focus on error reporting (Sprenger, 2001). The reporting system needs to be designed for learning, accountability, and redesign that prevents the likelihood the same error will reoccur (Tokarski, 2001). Too often, adjustment and correction of errors, if they occur, take place in a vacuum with only a select few individuals knowing about the incident (Sprenger, 2001). Sharing the experiences of the error or the factors that could have led to an error, facilitates an opportunity for learning that will only occur when the fear of punitive action is eliminated from within the health care environment, and positive rewards and recognition are given for quality improvement through redesigning a safer system.

THE COST OF ERRORS IN HEALTH CARE

The Institute of Medicine (IOM) 1999 report *To Err Is Human: Building a Safer Health System* indicated that between 44,000 and 98,000 people die each year as a result of medical errors (Kohn, Corrigan, & Donaldson, 2000). Medical errors rank as the eighth leading cause of death exceeding motor vehicle accidents, breast cancer, and AIDS. A 1998 report from the President's Advisory Commission on Consumer Protection and Quality in the Health Care Industry identified medical errors as one of the four major challenges in improving the quality of health care. The IOM report estimates that the cost of medical errors is in excess of $37 billion per year (Kohn, Corrigan, & Donaldson, 2000). Approximately half of this cost is associated with preventable errors. Additional costs include loss of trust by patients and families and diminished satisfaction for patients and health care professionals (Sprenger, 2001). Yet too often, silence continues to surround errors and practice breakdowns.

In the 2001 IOM report *Crossing the Quality Chasm* (Committee on Quality of Health Care in America, 2001), six aims for improving the quality of health care were identified: (1) patient safety, (2) patient centeredness; (3) effectiveness; (4) efficiency; (5) timeliness; and (6) equity. Patient safety without these six intertwined patient care goals cannot be achieved. Safe care also must be high-quality care. Also, the focus on quality must be based on continual experiential learning, assessment, reflection, and correction and redesign of care to improve the quality.

Research shows that most (70%) medical errors can be prevented (Agency for Healthcare Research and Quality [AHRQ], 2000). Most agree that recognizing and admitting errors and promoting improvement are far better strategies than denying the occurrence of the error or support of denial and cover-up through encouraging retribution and punitive sanctions (Kohn, et al, 2000). The best practices for preventing and managing errors continue to require research (Kizer, 2001).

NURSES AND PREVENTION

Nurses, because of their generalist education, continuous presence with patients, and tradition of patient advocacy, play a key role in the reduction of error in health care today (Benner et al., 2002). Nurses and nursing assistive staff comprise the majority of the health care providers. Patients have the most contact and spend the greatest amount of time with nurses. Patients and their families depend on nurses to provide safe care at a most vulnerable time in their lives. Vigilance and engagement in self-monitoring are continuously required yet are often overlooked factors that can prevent errors (Liolios, 2003). According to Borrell-Carrio and Epstein (2004), evidence suggests that errors do not often result from a lack of knowledge, but rather they occur because of "the mindless application of unexamined habits and the interference of unexamined emotions" (Borrell-Carrio & Epstein, 2004, p. 310).

Patient interactions with health care professionals are essential elements in the recognition and prevention of errors. Including the patient as a partner in health care may also increase patient safety. For example, if patients are aware of their own medical history and know the medications they are taking, and the medications to which they are allergic, they are better able to identify possible errors and injuries regarding their own health care than if they are not aware of and knowledgeable about these factors. Further, they may be able to actually intercept an error at some point in time and enhance their own safety (Weingart et al., 2005).

Kizer (2001) recommended that health care providers conduct self-assessments or audits to identify patient safety hazards and improve care processes. Examining prevention from a proactive rather than a reactive stance may strengthen the possibility of eliminating the punitive aspects and focus on root causes of errors.

Nurses learn early in their education the basic fundamentals of providing care. Prevention is so intertwined in nursing fundamentals that it is difficult at times to separate it. The increased demand on nurses has caused many nurses to function and work in an overload capacity, which ultimately may cause substandard patient care.

Often prevention becomes second nature and includes taking precautions to avoid infection, positioning patients, and other commonly practiced interventions. Jastremski, a registered nurse from Rome Memorial Hospital in Rome, New York, evaluated the occurrence of errors in the ICU. She noted that the simple task of hand washing may be omitted or done improperly because of increased demands, resulting in increased rates for nosocomial infections (Liolios, 2003).

Some examples of practice breakdown related to prevention include:

1. Not taking preventive measures to ensure patients' well-being. This includes lack of prevention of the hazards of immobility, such as skin breakdown, thrombus, muscle atrophy, kidney stones, and contractures.
2. Breach of infection precautions. This category can include use of contaminated equipment, not following isolation procedures, and not taking precautions for infection control.
3. Not providing a safe environment. This includes failure to ensure that equipment is safe prior to use, continued inappropriate use of equipment, and inadequate supervision or assistance.

PROTECTING SPECIFIC PATIENT VULNERABILITIES

Even under the best of circumstances, hospitalization presents hazards to patients. Much of nursing work has to do with ameliorating or preventing these hazards. The first class of hazards has to do with the vulnerabilities related to the patient's illness, disabilities, age, or cognitive functioning. For example, patients with cognitive impairments may not be able to request help adequately. Children's families must provide information about a child's daily routines, health status and growth pattern, medical history, preferences, and capacities. Infants, children, persons with disabilities, and the elderly require specific planning for communicating their needs and providing for their safety in a hospital. Patient safety requires specific planning and communication of specific potential hazards to prevent patients from falling, from receiving medications or foods that cause allergic responses, and from other hazards specific to particular patients.

THE HAZARDS OF PATIENT IMMOBILITY DURING HOSPITALIZATION

A second class of potential injuries relates to decreased mobility or immobility in patients who are bedridden. Nurses attend to the hazards of immobility, such as muscle contractions, stasis pneumonia, poor oral hygiene, and the risks of patient falls. Nutrition has to be monitored for patients with impairments that may prevent normal eating. A major challenge for elderly persons who are hospitalized is that they lose functional capacities that they had prior to hospitalization. For example, one week with little ambulation may require special interventions in assisting elderly patients to regain their ability to walk safely.

It is reported that 2.5 million patients are treated for pressure ulcers annually in the United States, and more than 50,000 patients die as a result of complications related to pressure ulcers (Ayello & Braden, 2002; Lyder, 2003; Reddy, Gill, & Rochon, 2006). Prevention of decubitus ulcers depends on many factors directly associated with *standard nursing interventions* aimed at preventing complications due to immobility, such as hygiene, hydration, electrolyte balance, nutrition, adequate and frequent positioning, use of support devices to protect patients' skin and bodies in bed, and more such hazards associated with particular patient morbidities related to bed rest and immobility.

Prevention of venous thromboembolism (VTE) requires attending to the risk factors for VTE, such as immobility, inactivity, specific disease processes such as cancer, nephrotic syndrome, heart failure, indwelling urinary catheters, and more (Wachter, 2008). Pulmonary embolism is especially dangerous to patients who are compromised by heart failure and other comorbidities. Autopsy studies have shown that almost half of the patients who die in the hospital will have had a pulmonary embolism, which is often undiagnosed prior to death (Shojania et al., 2003). The following risk factors for patient falls in the hospital (Currie, 2008) based on STRATIFY (St. Thomas Risk Assessment Tool in Falling Elderly Inpatients) are identified in Table 6.1.

Checklists are central to ensuring ongoing good and improving prevention in health care institutions (Gawande, 2007; Pronovost, Miller, & Wachter, 2006; Pronovost, Weast, & Rosenstein, 2005), and nurses are central to the

TABLE **6.1 Risk Factors for Patient Falls in the Hospital**

Fall as presenting complaint or history of falls
Mobility impairment or unstable gait
Muscle weakness
Use of assistive devices
Postural hypotension
Visual deficits
Cognitive impairment
Agitation
Urinary frequency
Medications (e.g., psychotropics, class Ia antiarrhythmics, digoxin, and diuretics)
Environmental factors (e.g., poor lighting, loose carpets)
Arthritis
Depression
Age greater than 80 years

From Bogardus, S.T. (2003). Risk factors for falls in the hospital. In: Another fall [Spotlight]. *AHRQ WebM&M* (Serial online). Available online at http://www.webnn.ahrq.gov.
See also: Agostini, J.V., Baker, D.I., Bogardus, S.T. (2001). *Prevention of falls in hospitalized and institutionalized older people*. Rockville, MD: The Agency for Healthcare Research and Quality.Currie, L. (2008). Fall and injury prevention. In Hughes R.G. (Ed.). *Patient safety and quality: An evidence-based handbook for nurses*. Rockville, MD: Agency for Healthcare Research and Quality. Available online at www.ahrq.gov/qual/nurseshdbk/. Accessed November 14, 2008.

effectiveness of implementing and maintaining adherence to checklists (Gawande, 2007). New efforts aimed at assessing risk factors for falls and prevention of decubitus ulcers and contractures now include preventive checklists. Maintaining functional status during hospitalization, especially for elderly patients, is impossible if the initial assessment of the patient's functional status is incomplete and the daily functional status is not checked against the initial functional status.

HOSPITAL-ACQUIRED INFECTIONS

A third class of hazards has to do with the dangers of hospital-acquired infections. The United States Centers for Disease Control and Prevention estimate that two million Americans develop infections while hospitalized, and of that number 90,000 die from those infections. Patients with immune problems are particularly at risk, but any patient may acquire an infection from breaks in sterile technique or from a lack of adequate hand washing on the part of the nurses and other health care workers. Some procedures such as continuous intravenous sites and drainage tubes such as urinary catheters, chest tubes, and nasogastric tubes require surveillance and specific interventions to lower the possibility of infections.

Hospital-wide efforts at reducing nosocomial infections have proved effective. For example, a study at Johns Hopkins Hospital showed a dramatic reduction in the number of bloodstream infections related to central venous catheters by strict adherence to a proven preventative protocol monitored by a checklist kept by nurses (Berenholtz et al., 2004; Gawande, 2007). Elements of the bundle of interventions to prevent central line infections included (1) hand hygiene, (2) maximal barrier precautions, (3) chlorhexidine skin antiseptics, (4) optimal catheter site selection with the subclavian vein as the preferred site for nontunneled catheters, and (5) daily review of the need for lines (using a checklist) with prompt removal of lines. It was also suggested that the femoral site of catheterization should be avoided if at all possible.

Urinary catheter infections account for about 40% of the hospital infections in the United States (Wachter, 2008). Patient factors that increase the risk of urinary catheter infections include duration of catheterization, patient age, and history of malignancy (Nicolle, 2005). Nurses can be instrumental in preventing the prolonged use of indwelling catheters, and system designs that give an automatic stop order for catheters have been shown to be helpful (Saint et al., 2006).

Preventing infections requires vigilance on the part of all health care workers. However, nurses take primary responsibility for establishing surveillance systems and preventive procedures such as rotation of intravenous sites, dressing changes, and general hygiene for patients. For example, routine lab work is checked daily to make sure that it is still necessary, and nurses have an informal maxim that if a technical intervention is not helping or needed, then it is potentially harmful to the patient.

Preventing errors is a systems issue as well as an individual nurse issue. Staffing levels play an important role in prevention. The AHRQ report, *Making Health Care Safer: A Critical Analysis of Patient Safety Practices* (2001), concludes that "leaner nurse staffing is associated with increased length of stay, nosocomial infection, and pressure ulcers" (p. 430). Needleman and colleagues (2002) found higher levels of staffing with registered nurses to be associated with lower rates of infection and gastrointestinal bleeding and shorter lengths of stay. Other systems issues include environmental factors such as workspace design, policies and procedures, and administrative support.

Most nurses do not intend to make errors or to injure patients at work. The perfectionist attitude of many nurses plays an important role in that health care professionals are expected to function without error (Sprenger, 2001). Error is viewed as failure. Yet, how can an acceptable error rate be identified and how can these errors be considered acceptable when people's lives are at stake? Some of the characteristics that are barriers to change include a tendency to view errors in several ways: (1) as a failure and deserving of blame; (2) as a difference in thinking that nursing emphasizes rules versus medicine's emphasis on knowledge; (3) as corrective actions that focus only on the individual versus looking at the entire health care team and system; and (4) as the thinking that assumes no harm has occurred if a patient is not injured (Tokarski, 2001). These barriers present many problem-solving activities and challenges, and yet hold the potential for changes in behavior and thinking.

Identifying, reducing, and ultimately preventing errors requires commitment and participation from the entire health care team including leadership and management. As Sprenger (2001) stated in his article "Sharing Responsibility for Patient Safety," a health care team is only as strong as its weakest link, and each of us needs to be accountable when an error occurs. Health care must acknowledge the seriousness of the errors and the shared responsibility necessary to address the problem (Kizer, 2001). In addition, a change in beliefs and practices from within a health care organization may be necessary in order to enhance quality and create a culture of safety that nurtures teamwork.

Surgical site infections can be dramatically reduced by four proven measures: (1) use of prophylactic antibiotics that are discontinued within 24 hours after surgery; (2) use of clippers instead of razors for hair removal prior to surgery; (3) maintaining tight glucose control; and (4) maintaining postoperative normothermia (Brennan et al., 1991; Mayhall, 2004; Melling et al., 2001; van den Berghe et al., 2001; Wenzel, 2002).

Ultimately, new ways of thinking may be necessary in order to address the challenges of improving patient safety as we know it today. The Veterans Administration Expert Panel on Patient Safety System Design (2001) recommended that health care organizations establish a voluntary reporting system that is nonpunitive and confidential in order to prevent errors and improve patient safety throughout their system (Tokarski, 2001). The work of nursing includes recognizing the importance of patient safety and prevention of nursing practice breakdown that leads to lack of prevention of known risks of immobility and hospitalization. Nursing efforts must now be enhanced by systematic and agreed-upon monitoring strategies, such as checklists with follow-through assessments of nurse-sensitive patient outcomes related to complications due to hospitalization and immobility and known patient risk factors.

HISTORICAL CASE STUDY #1: An Ounce of Prevention

PRACTICE BREAKDOWN AND PREVENTION

BACKGROUND

An outpatient oncology clinic was located in a small town with a population of approximately 20,000. The clinic had been open for approximately 5 years. Dr. Dave Brown owned the clinic, and the local hospital had provided financial assistance to start the clinic.

Ms. Danielle Davis, RN, had been employed by Dr. Brown prior to the opening of the clinic. The state board of nursing received a complaint that Nurse Davis was engaging in unsafe practices.

THE NURSE'S STORY

Nurse Davis had been licensed as a registered nurse for 20 years during which time she had worked primarily in the hospital setting on the medical-surgical, coronary care, and intensive care units and in the emergency department. She accepted an offer from Dr. Brown to work as a nurse in the oncology clinic.

Nurse Davis informed Dr. Brown that she had no experience in oncology nursing. Dr. Brown assured her that he would provide her with training. He did train Nurse Davis in oncology treatment practices before she began working with patients. Her duties included administering chemotherapy, preparing medications and chemotherapy agents, accessing ports, drawing blood from ports, flushing ports, administering medications through the ports, and following proper infection control practices and procedures. Dr. Brown said that he had observed her frequently during her employment at the clinic.

The clinic had applied to participate in oncology clinical trials. A registered nurse consultant, Ms. Connie Cousins, came to the clinic to conduct an on-site inspection and evaluation. Consultant Cousins observed many substandard practices while at the clinic. She shared her report with Nurse Davis and with Dr. Brown. Dr. Brown asked that Consultant Nurse Cousins refrain from providing a copy of the report to the local hospital, but Consultant Nurse Cousins ignored this request and provided a copy of the report to the hospital.

Some of the observed substandard practices that failed to follow basic infection control requirements when providing treatment included the following:

1. Reusing single-use disposable syringes from the same patient when accessing a bag of saline that was used for multiple patients.

2. Injecting patient's blood back into the patient's port after drawing blood for lab testing.
3. Reusing syringes to mix multiple chemotherapeutic agents.
4. Storing admixed medications in the drug cabinet for future patient use without labeling the medications with the time and date the medication was mixed.
5. Failing to label IV bags or syringes with the patient's name and the contents of the bag.
6. Maintaining food and food supplies in the same cabinet as the chemotherapy medications.
7. Discarding chemotherapy-contaminated supplies in the regular trash container.
8. Failing to wear gloves when providing care for patients.

ADDITIONAL INFORMATION

Ms. Joan Deming, a trained dental hygienist, was employed as a receptionist at the oncology clinic. She informed Dr. Brown on at least one occasion that she had observed Nurse Davis and the other registered nurses employed at the clinic engaging in improper infection control practices.

Ms. Brigette Ingersol was a registered nurse who worked as the infection control registered nurse at the local hospital. Several patients from the oncology clinic approached her with concerns about practices at the clinic. These practices included reusing syringes that had been used to draw blood to obtain saline from a large saline bag, then using the saline to flush patients' ports.

Consultant Nurse Cousins' report concluded that the nurses were unable to develop a correction plan regarding the observed unsafe practices. She indicated the part-time registered nurses were overwhelmed with information and that Nurse Davis appeared unwilling to discuss options to correct the practices.

Mr. Niles Anderson became a patient of the clinic. Mr. Anderson was positive for the hepatitis C virus (HCV). He received blood draws and chemotherapy at the clinic. Approximately 1 year after he became a patient, Mr. Walter Belin, another patient, was diagnosed with HCV. Two weeks later, Mr. Tony Caruthers, a third patient, was diagnosed with HCV. Both Mr. Belin and Mr. Carruthers were diagnosed with HCV approximately 2 months prior to Consultant Nurse Cousins' visit to the clinic.

One month after Consultant Nurse Cousins' visit, Nurse Ingersol met with Dr. Brown to discuss ongoing concerns expressed to her by several clinic patients regarding unsafe practices at the clinic. In the next 2 weeks, Mr. John Dickson and Mr. Dan Edison, both clinic patients, were diagnosed with HCV. Shortly after the diagnosis of Mr. Dickson and Mr. Edison, Nurse Davis resigned. In the next year, 100 clinic patients were diagnosed with HCV. Of that number, three died as a result of the HCV infection.

The board of nursing reviewed Nurse Davis' case and recommended revocation of her registered nurse license. The license was revoked.

CASE ANALYSIS

Infection control precautions are basic to the health care profession. Safe practices are the foundation of any procedure or task. In this case, many individuals either did not maintain basic infection control procedures or were unaware that the proper precautions were not being followed. Lack of training and certification in chemotherapy medication administration also contributed to the nurses' lack of knowledge and skill.

Nurse Davis was the full-time registered nurse at the clinic and carried responsibility for care practices of the other staff at the clinic. She did not practice basic infection control and was not aware that others were not following infection control measures.

The physician was aware of and routinely observed unsafe practices in his clinic. The nurse consultant, the registered nurse, and the infection control nurse at the hospital had made both the physician and his employee, the registered nurse, aware of the unsafe practices being conducted at the clinic.

This is a case where the use of simple infection control precautions could have prevented many individuals from becoming infected with HCV and could have prevented the death and suffering of patients in this vulnerable patient population.

References

Agency for Healthcare Research and Quality (AHRQ). (2000). *Medical errors: The scope of the problem.* Rockville, MD: AHRQ. (Publication No. AHRQ 00-P037). Available online at http://www.ahrq.gov/qual/errback.htm. Accessed October 2, 2008.

Agency for Healthcare Research and Quality (AHRQ). (2001). *Making health care safer: A critical analysis of patient safety practices.* Rockville, MD: AHRQ. (Publication No. AHRQ 01-E058). Available online at http://www.ahrq.gov/clinic/ptsafety/. Accessed October 2, 2008.

Ayello, E. A., & Braden, B. (2002). How and why to do pressure ulcer risk assessment. *Advances in Skin & Wound Care, 15*(3), 125-131.

Benner, P., Sheets, V., Uris, P., Malloch, K., Schwed, K., & Jamison, D. (2002). Individual, practice, and system causes of errors in nursing: A taxonomy. *Journal of Nursing Administration, 32*(10), 509-523.

Berenholtz, S. M., Pronovost, P. J., Lipsett, P. A., Hobson, D., Earsing, K., Farley, J. E., et al. (2004). Eliminating catheter-related bloodstream infections in the intensive care unit. *Critical Care Medicine, 32*(10), 2014-2020.

Bogardus, S. T. (2003). Risk factors for falls in the hospital. In: Another fall [Spotlight]. *AHRQ WebM&M* (Serial online). Available online at http://www.webmm.ahrq.gov. Accessed November 14, 2008.

Borrell-Carrio, F., & Epstein, R. M. (2004). Preventing errors in clinical practice: A call for self awareness. *Annals of Family Medicine, 2*(4), 310-316.

Brennan, T. A., Leape, L. L., Laird, N. M., Hebert, L., Localio, A. R., Lawthers, A. G., et al. (1991). Incidence of adverse events and negligence in hospitalized patients. Results of the Harvard Medical Practice Study I. *New England Journal of Medicine, 324*(6), 370-376.

Committee on Quality of Health Care in America, Institute of Medicine. (2001). *Crossing the quality chasm: A new health system for the 21st century*. Washington, DC: The National Academies Press.

Currie, L. (2008). Fall and injury prevention. In R. G. Hughes (Ed.), *Patient safety and quality: An evidence-based handbook for nurses*. Rockville, MD: Agency for Healthcare Research and Quality. Available online at www.ahrq.gov/qual/nurseshdbk/. Accessed November 14, 2008.

Gawande, A. (2007). Annals of Medicine: The Checklist. If something so simple can transform intensive care, what else can it do? *The New Yorker*, December 10, 2007.

Kizer, K. W. (2001). Patient safety: A call to action: A consensus statement from the National Quality Forum. *Medscape General Medicine, 3*(2), 10.

Kohn, L. T., Corrigan, J. M., & Donaldson, M. S. (Eds.); Committee on Quality of Health Care in America, Institute of Medicine. (2000). *To err is human: Building a safer health system*. Washington, D.C.: The National Academies Press.

Liolios, A. (2003). Looking at various perspectives, researchers seek to reduce errors in the ICU. *Abstracts of the 32nd Critical Care Congress of the Society of Critical Care Medicine*. Available online at www.medscape.com. Accessed October 2, 2008.

Lyder, C. H. (2003). Pressure ulcer prevention and management. *Journal of the American Medical Association, 289*(2), 223-226.

National Council of State Boards of Nursing (NCSBN). (2006). *TERCAP protocol*. Available online at http//www.NCSBN.org. Accessed November 17, 2008.

Marx, D. (2001). *Patient safety and the "just culture": A primer for health care executives*. New York: Columbia University Press.

Mayhall, G. (2004). *Hospital epidemiology and infection control* (3rd ed.). Philadelphia: Lippincott Williams & Wilkins.

Melling, A. C., Ali, B., Scott, E. M., & Leaper, D. J. (2001). Effects of preoperative warming on the incidence of wound infection after clean surgery: A randomised controlled trial. *Lancet, 358*(9285), 876-880.

Needleman, J., Buerhaus, P., Mattke, S., Stewart, M., & Zelevinsky, K. (2002). Nurse-staffing levels and the quality of care in hospitals. *New England Journal of Medicine, 346*(22), 1715-1722.

Nicolle, L. E. (2005). Catheter-related urinary tract infections. *Drugs & Aging, 22*(8), 627-639.

President's Advisory Commission on Consumer Protection and Quality in the Health Care Industry. (1998). Quality first: Better health care for all Americans. Available online at http://www.hcqualitycommission.gov/final. Accessed October 2, 2008.

Pronovost, P., Weast, B., & Rosenstein, B. (2005). Implementing and validating a comprehensive unit-based safety program. *Journal of Patient Safety, 1*, 33-40.

Pronovost, P. J., Miller, M. R., & Wachter, R. M. (2006). Tracking progress in patient safety: An elusive target. *Journal of the American Medical Association, 296*(6), 696-699.

Reddy, M., Gill, S. S., & Rochon, P. A. (2006). Preventing pressure ulcers: A systematic review. *Journal of the American Medical Association, 296*(8), 974-984.

Saint, S., Kaufman, S. R., Rogers, M. A., Baker, P. D., Ossenkop, K., & Lipsky, B. A. (2006). Condom versus indwelling urinary catheters: A randomized trial. *Journal of the American Geriatrics Society, 54*(7), 1055-1061.

Shojania, K. G., Burton, E. C., McDonald, K. M., & Goldman, L. (2003). Changes in rates of autopsy-detected diagnostic errors over time: A systematic review. *Journal of the American Medical Association, 289*(21), 2849-2856.

Sprenger, G. (2001). Sharing responsibility for patient safety. *American Journal of Health-System Pharmacy, 58*(11), 988-989.

Tokarski, C. (2001). Effective practices: Improve patient safety summit. *Medscape.* Retrieved October 19, 2005, from www.medscape.com

van den Berghe, G., Wouters, P., Weekers, F., Verwaest, C., Bruyninckx, F., Schetz, M., et al. (2001). Intensive insulin therapy in the critically ill patients. *New England Journal of Medicine, 345*(19), 1359-1367.

Wachter, R. M. (2008). *Understanding patient safety.* New York: McGraw Hill Medical.

Weingart, S. N., Pagovich, O., Sands, D. Z., Li, J. M., Aronson, M. D., Davis, R. B., et al. (2005). What can hospitalized patients tell us about adverse events? Learning from patient-reported incidents. *Journal of General Internal Medicine, 20*(9), 830-836.

Wenzel, R. P. (2002). *Prevention and control of nosocomial infections* (4th ed.). Philadelphia: Lippincott Williams & Wilkins.

7

Practice Breakdown: Intervention

Mary Beth Thomas ◆ *Patricia Benner*

Chapter Outline

CAREGIVING PRACTICES: A FRAMEWORK FOR NURSING INTERVENTIONS

TERCAP® includes a practice breakdown category entitled "Intervening," which indicates that a nurse *acts* correctly on behalf of a patient. A practice breakdown in intervention presents a challenge with the *execution* and *timing* of a nursing action and *not* with clinical discernment and reasoning or with a decision to initiate an intervention. Selecting and initiating the interventions would be considered a breakdown in diagnostic discernment or clinical reasoning. Many of the preventive measures for patient safety are standard nursing interventions, but two separate categories are needed since "prevention" only shows up as an error when it is absent or faulty in some way. Interventions such as "using the least restrictive type of restraints for patient safety" can show up as ill-chosen or poorly or mistakenly done. The range of nursing interventions, of course, extends beyond preventive nursing interventions, to any therapeutic interventions, psychosocial interventions, comfort measures, educational interventions, and more.

Intervention, as defined in TERCAP, does *not* include nursing assessments, surveillance, and monitoring. These aspects of nursing practice are captured under other TERCAP categories. However, assessment, surveillance, and monitoring provide the foundation for effective nursing interventions that are implemented to promote patient well-being and prevent hazards inherent in immobilization and hospitalization.

INTERVENTIONS WITHIN A CONTEXT OF CARING

Nurses provide interventions to assist patients in reaching mutually expected goals and/or outcomes based on established ethical, professional, and legal relationships. Some of these interventions are unique to the nursing profession and are established within a framework of caring or caring practices.

Caring may be defined as sentiment, as in the human expression of respect for and response to wholeness. We locate sentiments associated with caring within public caregiving practices rather than in private experiences. In this definition of caring and caregiving, nursing is a socially organized practice with notions of *good* internal to the practice (Dunne, 1993; MacIntyre, 1984). Caring is also defined as a part of perceptual and cognitive capacities as in personal, empirical, ethical, and aesthetic ways of knowing (Boykin & Schoenhofer, 1990). Caring about a patient's well-being and protecting the vulnerabilities of clients or patients are at the heart of the nursing tradition and are central to nursing practice. In this regard, caring and caregiving are defined as caring *practices* and comprise a range of nursing interventions.

Nursing interventions are what nurses "do." Scholars and practitioners have developed nursing intervention classification systems to outline and standardize common nursing interventions as a means to promote communication and understanding of what nurses do. These bodies of information present a taxonomy or classification of nursing work based on commonly held agreements on central expectations of good practice in nursing.

Florence Nightingale was the first nurse to develop a classification system to organize thinking and notions of public health and health promotion. She advanced our understanding of an individual's inherent physical capacity to resist infection, heal, and recover. Nightingale was concerned about the environment and about placing the body in the best conditions in which to heal.

Intervention classification systems have expanded as professionalism in nursing has evolved over the years. Currently there are several nursing classification systems reflecting different theoretical approaches to naming what nurses do (Gordon, 1998). These have led to discourse and disagreement within the profession, and these debates continue to underscore the richness and diversity of the work in nursing formulated through an assessment of signs, symptoms, and diagnosis of a patient's condition and responses. They are deliberate and knowledge based and skill based in that the nurse continuously evaluates nuances in the patient's response to interventions and adjusts future interventions accordingly (Benner, 1984; 2001).

Nurses develop perceptual capacities that enable them to recognize and intervene when a patient's recovery or clinical condition is not usual or as expected. Often this recognition comes as a gestalt of the way that a patient appears, the cluster of evolving vital signs, or a tacit comparison with other patients with similar conditions. This perceptual acuity based on past experiences with similar patients is characterized as an intuitive aspect in recognizing the need for more assessment and/or intervention. The intuitive aspect refers to the tacit, experience-based expectations and perceptual capacities that the nurse develops over time as a result of seeing and caring for many patients. Attentiveness and observation across time are paramount in this process because of the patient who may change from moment to moment (see Chapter 4).

VISIBLE AND INVISIBLE NURSING ACTIVITIES

Nursing activities can be both visible and invisible (Page, 2004; Star & Strauss, 1999). The foundation for providing appropriate and timely nursing interventions includes accounting for and prioritizing both visible and invisible nursing practices.

Visible activities are easily observed by the public. Administering treatments, educating patients, and intervening with other health care providers are all activities that when observed are easy to identify and understand. However, even these visible activities may occur in the privacy of a patient's room and might not be observed by others.

Ongoing core components of nursing practice include the nursing processes of assessment, surveillance, coordination of care, and other cognitive activities that are less visible and not as easy to observe. These invisible nursing assessments make safe and timely interventions possible. These aspects of nursing practice are identified as "monitoring, surveillance, and attentiveness," (Chapter 4) and constitute the background for intelligent, well-timed, nursing interventions.

INTERVENTIONS TO PROTECT PATIENT VULNERABILITIES

Nurses are the professionals at the "sharp end" of patient care (Page, 2004). Nurses are present 24 hours a day, 7 days a week, and much of their work requires timely interventions. Nurses deliver most of the prescribed therapies for patient care. Nursing interventions have become more central to patient safety partly because hospitalized patients are sicker and require adjusting therapies to the patient's particular response. Aiken (2005) notes:

> Patients may have more than one surgical site, multiple monitors, an artificial respirator, and an intravenous line administering powerful drugs that can result in death if the infusion rate is not correct. On average, nurses care for 5 to 6 postoperative patients at a time. Everyday, about one third of nurses' patients arrive directly from the operating room or are admitted in acute medical crises. One third are in the early stages of recovery or stabilization, with many requirements for nursing time and one third are being discharged, often with complicated home care requirements (p. 180).

Nurses develop communication systems and patient care plans to ensure that nursing interventions are implemented in an accurate and timely manner. Planned nursing interventions are governed by patients' therapies and treatment. However, many nursing interventions are required to protect patients from both internal and external vulnerabilities. For example, when patients cannot ambulate, they must be protected from hazards of immobility, such as decubitus ulcers, contractures, stasis pneumonia, falls, or infections (Steed, 1999). In addition, many patients' vulnerabilities, such as cognitive impairment, impaired mobility, drowsiness, or dizziness, require additional nursing precautions to prevent patient falls and poor hygiene and to promote proper toileting and other daily functions of living. Such nursing interventions are expected and are necessary for patient safety in the hospital. Substandard nursing care includes lack of nursing interventions regarding these vulnerabilities, impairments, predictable activities of daily living, and safety precautions. These interventions usually show up, as noted above, as lack of prevention.

EXTERNAL THREATS TO PATIENT SAFETY

Threats to patient safety, such as errors perpetuated by a large health care system, necessitate that management and nursing staff develop surveillance systems for patient safety. Activities that promote patient safety, such as preventing hospital-acquired infections, are usually integrated into the quality assurance programs of hospitals. We have also considered the practice breakdown category of lack of preventive interventions. Researchers have recently examined the importance of staffing and its impact on patient safety (Blegen, Good, & Reed, 1998; Buerhaus et al., 2002; Clarke, Sloane, & Aiken, 2002). Planning for adequate nursing care is evaluated through staffing ratios determined by patient care needs. Higher patient acuity or complex care patients require more nursing care and surveillance and, ideally, nurse-patient ratios are adjusted accordingly.

PATIENT-RELATED VULNERABILITIES

The Practice Breakdown Advisory Panel found that patients with cognitive or sensory impairments were at greater risk for practice breakdown, suggesting that a higher nurse-to-patient ratio is also needed for these patients. Examining incidents of practice breakdown can assist with improving the design of the infrastructures related to promoting patient safety.

Safe and accurate nursing interventions depend on adequate patient monitoring, adequate planned safety measures to match patients' specific needs, and good clinical judgment (Benner, Hooper-Kyriakidis, & Stannard, 1999). Much of the safety work of nurses is taken for granted because it is so pervasive and essential to patient well-being.

The following is an overview of important patient vulnerabilities that require examination to ensure appropriate and adequate nursing interventions:

1. Interventions to Protect Patients From Vulnerabilities Due to Illness, Disability, Age, and Cognition. Even under the best of circumstances, hospitalization may present potential hazards to patients. Much of the work of nursing has to do with ameliorating or preventing these hazards. The first class of hazards points to the vulnerabilities related to the patient's illness, disabilities, age, or cognitive functioning. For example, patients with cognitive impairments may not be able to make adequate requests for help, or a family with an ill child must provide information about the child's daily routines, medical history, preferences, and capacities without which gaps occur in medical treatment and nursing care. Frail elderly persons, infants, children, and persons with disabilities require specific planning to communicate their needs and provide for their safety in the hospital. Individualized measures for patient safety require planning and communication of potential hazards to prevent patients from falling, from receiving medications or foods that cause allergic responses, and from many other hazards specific to particular patients.

2. *Interventions to Prevent the Hazards of Patient Immobility.* A second class of potential injuries relates to decreased mobility or immobility in patients who are bedridden (Olson, 1967). Nurses intervene to prevent the hazards of immobility such as muscle contractions, stasis pneumonia, poor oral hygiene, and risks of patient falls. Patients with impairments that prevent normal eating need monitoring to provide adequate nutrition. Poorly timed or selected interventions to prevent patient safety hazards typically show up as lack of preventive measures. Typically, when errors of "omission" occur (such as a lack of intervention in potential patient safety hazards) (see Chapter 6), they are discovered in patient outcomes when it is too late to prevent the hazard. For example, a patient may develop "foot drop" when exercises, ambulation, footboards, or splints are not used early in the patient's care. Consequently, on the TERCAP tool, the Prevention and Intervention categories are often both chosen as the major "types" of errors.

A major nursing goal in the care of elderly persons is to maintain or increase the functional capacities that they had on admission to the hospital. If specific nursing interventions are not undertaken, elderly patients will frequently lose the functional capacities that they had prior to hospital admission. For example, as little as one week with minimal ambulation may require special interventions in assisting elderly patients to regain the ability to walk safely. Loss of bladder control can be a major deleterious outcome of hospitalization or any institutionalization of older patients.

Clearly, even with timely nursing interventions to prevent immobility, all hazards may not be prevented in all patients. For example, a patient may be too unstable physiologically (e.g., because of compromised hemodynamics), or even psychologically, to complete all of the physical therapy that would be required to prevent muscle wasting.

Improved technologies have been developed to help prevent hazards of immobility. For instance, specialized beds that alternate pressure points and assist with patient positioning have been implemented to improve the care of comatose patients. Nurses have demonstrated the effectiveness of nursing measures to prevent most of the hazards of immobility most of the time for most patients. For example, the incidence of pneumonia for patients on ventilators has decreased dramatically with nursing interventions of hand hygiene, frequent and effective mouth care, and patient positioning (Hsieh & Tuite, 2006).

3. *Interventions to Prevent Nosocomial Infections.* A third class of hazards has to do with the dangers of nosocomial infections. Patients who are immunocompromised are particularly at risk, but any patient may acquire an infection from

breaks in sterile technique or from lack of or inadequate hand washing on the part of nurses and other health care workers. Some procedures that use continuous intravenous fluids, drainage tubes (such as urinary catheters), chest tubes, and nasogastric tubes require monitoring and specific interventions to lower the possibility for infections.

Preventing infections requires vigilance on the part of all health care workers; however, nurses have a primary responsibility in designing and implementing surveillance systems and preventive procedures, such as rotation of intravenous sites, dressing changes, and general hygiene for patients. For example, routine lab work is checked daily to determine whether it is still necessary. Nurses share an informal maxim that if a technical intervention is not helping or needed, then it is potentially harmful to the patient (Benner, Kyriakidis-Hooper, & Stannard, 1999).

4. Interventions to Prevent the Hazards of Technology. A fourth class of potential threats to patient safety has to do with the hazards of technology, such as the potential for electrical shock, malfunctioning equipment, or even inadequate supplies and equipment (Benner, Hooper-Kyriakides, & Stannard, 1999). Nurses play an integral role in the safety work required for preventing and maintaining infrastructures that monitor and intervene with potential hazards in highly technical health care environments.

Surgical patients are all at risk for hypothermia, inadequate grounding of electrical equipment, inadequate securing and positioning, and all of the potential hazards that occur when a patient is unconscious and is not able to withdraw from painful stimuli or complain of pain.

One of the cases reported to a state board involved inadequate securing of the patient on an operating room table. The patient fell to the floor during the surgery, breaking all sterile techniques. Fortunately, measures were taken to treat the patient's potential infection, no broken bones or major tissue injury occurred, and the patient recovered satisfactorily. Full disclosure was made to the patient and family soon after the surgery.

5. Interventions to Rescue Patients and Problems With Failure to Rescue Patients. Aiken and colleagues (2003) have used "failure to rescue" as a measure to assess the effectiveness of medical treatment and nursing care. Failure to rescue reflects a belief that institutional and staff resources can prevent or intercept patient catastrophes. These resources involve surveillance and effective rescue interventions (Clarke & Aiken, 2003) (see Chapter 4) for monitoring and recognizing the need for intervention. This combination of attentiveness and effective nursing interventions provides an essential foundation for safeguarding patients who may have compromised defense mechanisms due to illness and institutionalization.

Earlier, Aiken, Smith, and Lake (1994) conducted an epidemiologic study to evaluate the impact of nursing care on patient outcomes. They matched 195 control hospitals with 39 original magnet hospitals. The magnet hospitals had been formally evaluated and recognized for their quality of nursing care. The investigators used propensity scoring, a multivariate, matched sampling procedure that controlled for size, teaching status, technology, proportion of board-certified physicians, and selected hospital characteristics.

They found a 4.5% lower Medicare mortality rate in the magnet hospitals compared to the control hospitals not identified for their high quality of nursing care. They concluded that the quality of nursing care interventions has an impact on patient mortality and that failure to intervene appropriately to rescue patients in extreme circumstances contributed significantly to higher mortality rates in the control hospitals.

HISTORICAL CASE STUDY #1: Restraints Gone Awry

PRACTICE BREAKDOWN, INTERVENING

HISTORY

The following nursing activities and behaviors outlined in this case scenario provide an example of events that demonstrate a nurse's failure to intervene on behalf of her patient.

THE COMPLAINT

Ms. Maggie Jones was a registered nurse who worked in a prison setting. She was reported to the board of nursing through a complaint received as follow-up to the findings of a peer review committee. The committee determined that Nurse Jones exposed an inmate to risk of harm because of failure to adequately care for him.

In summary, the specific allegations indicated that Nurse Jones failed to conduct a thorough assessment of the inmate, continually evaluate and observe him, recognize early signs of his symptoms of respiratory compromise, and initiate life-saving measures. The committee concluded that Nurse Jones exhibited an inability to supervise and lead subordinates in cardiopulmonary resuscitation, which resulted in the inmate's death.

INVESTIGATION

An autopsy of the inmate showed mild hemorrhage in the soft tissues anterior to the larynx, severe congestion of the conjunctival and scleral vessels, severe congestion of the lungs, and petechiae on the epicardial surface of the heart. The pathologist determined that the inmate's death was caused by positional asphyxia. These conclusions were based on the autopsy findings and the events that were documented in a recorded video.

This incident involved a state prison inmate, Mr. Jimmy X, who had a history of attempted suicide through hanging. Mr. X had succeeded in hanging himself from the ceiling on the night of the reported incident but was quickly taken down and transported by gurney to the prison emergency room.

Once in the emergency room, Mr. X began to struggle. The staff decided to restrain him and place him prone with his legs brought up and secured close to his buttocks. Mr. X continued to struggle and started moaning after which he quickly became unresponsive to the staff. Security staff became concerned about

Mr. X's lack of movement and summoned medical assistance. A code was initiated, but Mr. X did not respond and died from positional asphyxia.

Nurse Jones had been assigned as charge nurse for the prison night shift. On the night of the incident, she was expected to orient Mr. Paul Phillips, a newly hired registered nurse who had been licensed for only 3 months. He was in his second month of practice at the facility. When the restrained inmate appeared to be in distress, Nurse Jones told Nurse Phillips to stay with the patient while she left the area to make "necessary calls."

Facility policy indicated that the charge nurse's duties included orientation of new staff, which was a role Nurse Jones had engaged in many times. A position description provided by the prison indicated that a nurse is the first health care provider to see an inmate and assess his/her health status to determine whether he/she is sick or malingering. Interviews with several staff members revealed that the culture of the prison led nurses to believe that they must always be cognizant of security needs and could not stop security personnel from using force.

Nurse Phillips stated that he had been licensed for only 3 months and had worked for the prison for only 2 months prior to the incident. Nurse Jones was assigned to be his preceptor that night. He had briefly been involved with an assessment of the inmate when he was first brought to the emergency room. The incident was his first code. He had never initiated CPR, but he did so because no one else was aiding Mr. X. He said he had called Nurse Jones but said that she left him shortly after arriving in the emergency room. Mr. Phillips reported that he felt that Nurse Jones did not take charge or provide him with any guidance during the episode. He continued CPR until he was relieved by paramedics.

Nurse Jones's statement was that she had excellent evaluations, good nursing assessment skills, and had never been counseled for job performance issues. She considered the code to be an unusual situation. The "hogtie" restraint that was used on Mr. X was routinely used by security as a means of restraint. She stated that, in her opinion, a reasonably prudent correctional nurse would not have foreseen that Mr. X would suffer positional asphyxia. When it was apparent that the patient was in trouble, she made the necessary calls to obtain assistance.

Nurse Jones indicated that she did not have Advanced Cardiac Life Support (ACLS) certification and did not have a current CPR certificate. Initiating CPR was not second nature to her. However, she considered herself an advocate for the patient. In fact, she had been moved from second shift to the night shift because she was characterized by her supervisors as being "weak," as evidenced by her "seeing the patients more times than was warranted." Nurse Jones' statement that her record was "unblemished" seems incongruent with her additional comment that she was moved from second shift because she was "weak and seeing inmates too many times."

Nurse Jones' actions demonstrated that she had no awareness of the possibility of post-trauma swelling and edema that could compromise breathing and that this possibility would not be immediately observable without an appropriate assessment. This lack of awareness constituted a major knowledge deficit. In this instance, the posthanging injury and the hogtie restraint placed the patient at risk for asphyxiation. The cause of death, according to the autopsy, was positional asphyxia, not injury from the attempted hanging. It is important to note that Nurse Jones did not take a leadership role in the code and attributed this to her lack of experience. During the investigation, it was found that Nurse Jones had been a licensed practical nurse for many years. Once in the emergency situation, Nurse Jones did not take the lead during the resuscitation attempt, which is the expected standard for her level and experience. Mr. Phillips, the recent registered nurse graduate and new employee, was left to his own resources without appropriate and necessary assistance.

ANALYSIS USING TERCAP: HEALTH CARE TEAM

Because the circumstances suggest a cavalier attitude by all persons involved, it is troublesome that Nurse Jones was the only individual singled out for discipline. This is an oversight in the investigation as other staff members' roles in this incident may have been at issue here. For instance, one question that arises is whether a well-defined process for medical emergencies was in place with physician oversight and review. Correctional facilities should have protocols in place to address these types of emergency issues. Additionally, questions arise as to the nurse's responsibility and authority in relation to security personnel. This case clearly demonstrates that nursing interventions should have been the priority and that the nurse should have had the organizationally mandated authority to direct the safety of the inmate's handling by the security guards.

Other team factors should have been investigated and additional questions asked including the following: What supervisory feedback had been provided to Nurse Jones? Should she have been put in a preceptor role? What is the culture for incorporating new graduates into autonomous staff positions? One must question the ways in which this incident affected the junior registered nurse as a newly graduated nurse. Clearly, more support and training should have been planned for his orientation on the job. This case also raises an important question related to continued competency, that is, What is the best way to ensure that nurses are both knowledgeable and capable of performing a seldom needed but extremely critical function?

ANALYSIS USING TERCAP: HEALTH CARE SYSTEM

Planning and training were issues in this scenario. Trauma and attempted hangings are anticipated events in a prison environment. Thus it is critical to ensure prior identification of these potential incidents with prepared emergency plans, training, and evaluation. Practicing through mock incidents is one of several approaches to address readiness. In addition, training for ACLS is needed given the requirements for resuscitation in a prison environment. In this regard, leadership should ensure inclusion of these training elements. Recognition of the emergency and intervening with basic airway/CPR techniques would likely have stabilized the inmate until EMS arrived. Given the prevalence of security personnel, they too should have been prepared to provide basic rescue interventions in situations of violence and injury.

The guards' behavior and training are also in question. Prior to this case, it appears that no one had questioned the procedure of restraining a person by means of a hogtie prone position, which was the direct cause of the inmate's suffocation in this incident. Such ties have been identified as unsafe and should be eliminated as a restraining measure. All personnel should be trained to adhere to restraint procedures that are safe and updated regularly.

Even though this was a prison setting, potential safety issues such as use of restraints for an injured inmate should have been implemented and directed by appropriate health care personnel. Additionally, there should have been a clear understanding of the hierarchy of authority and an identification of those in charge in this correctional facility.

AGGRESSIVE BEHAVIOR: PROTECTING THE PATIENT AND PROTECTING THE NURSE

The preceding case study reviews issues in caring for patients who demonstrate aggressive behavior. Caring for patients who exhibit aggressive behaviors is not limited to prison settings but rather transcends practice settings and population groups. For example, behavioral manifestations of aggression may range from elderly patients who become confused and disoriented after a surgical procedure to adolescents who are dealing with role identity and anger management issues to patients who experience a psychotic episode. Aggressive behavior can occur in any health care setting, and nurses must be prepared with specific interventions to ensure the safety of patients and staff.

When aggression is a component of patient behavior, the provision of nursing care becomes highly complex and may quickly lead to a dangerous situation. Practice breakdown can be exacerbated by the crisis that may occur with combative patients. Although the nurse should consider his/her own well-being and desire for safety, the urgent needs of the patient must be addressed. The nurse may have to manage the patient's attempt to harm others as well as protect the patient from self-harm. In addition, the nurse's duty to the patient may be compounded by other obligations, such as ensuring the safety of other patients or staff. This complex patient care situation can easily contribute to practice breakdown. The need for comprehensive planning and education cannot be overstated.

Some nursing disciplines are more prepared for aggression than others. For example, most psychiatric facilities have extensive training and protocols for preventing and managing aggressive behavior. Other settings may not have specific orientation or protocols to provide nurses with the education needed to address aggressive behaviors in specific workplace environments. Nurses must understand the etiology of and reasons for aggressive behavior in given patient populations and in particular practice settings, and protocols should reflect appropriate methods for recognizing and managing aggressive behavior. Finally, all institutions where resuscitation does not occur often must institute ongoing classes for health care personnel to ensure that nurses are prepared to provide effective and safe immediate rescue efforts for patients.

References

Aiken, L. H., Smith, H. L., & Lake, E. T. (1994). Lower Medicare mortality among a set of hospitals known for good nursing care. *Medical Care, 32*(8), 771-787.

Aiken, L. H., Clarke, S. P., Cheung, R. B., Sloane, D. M., & Silber, J. H. (2003). Education levels of hospital nurses and patient mortality. *Journal of the American Medical Association, 290*(12), 1617-1623.

Aiken, L. H. (2005). Improving quality through nursing. In D. Mechanic, L. B. Rogut, & D. C. Colby (Eds.), *Policy challenges in modern health care* (pp. 177-188). New Brunswick, NJ: Rutgers University Press.

Benner, P. (1984, 2001). *From novice to expert: Excellence and power in clinical nursing practice* (1st and 2nd ed.). Upper Saddle River, NJ: Prentice-Hall.

Benner, P., Hooper-Kyriakidis, P., & Stannard, D. (1999). *Clinical wisdom and interventions in critical care: A thinking-in-action approach.* Philadelphia: W.B. Saunders.

Blegen, M. A., Goode, C. J., & Reed, L. (1998). Nurse staffing and patient outcomes. *Nursing Research, 47*(1), 43-50.

Boykin, A., & Schoenhofer, S. (1990). Caring in nursing: Analysis of extant theory. *Nursing Science Quarterly, 3*(4), 149-155.

Buerhaus, P. I., Needleman, J., Mattke, S., & Stewart, M. (2002). Strengthening hospital nursing. *Health Affairs, 21*(5), 123-132.

Clarke, S. P., & Aiken, L. H. (2003). Failure to rescue. *American Journal of Nursing, 103* (1), 42-47.

Clarke, S. P., Sloane, D. M., & Aiken, L. H. (2002). The effects of hospital staffing and organizational climate on needle stick injuries to nurses. *American Journal of Public Health, 92*(7), 1115-1119.

Dunne, J. (1993). *Back to the rough ground: Practical judgment and the lure of technique.* Notre Dame, IN: University of Notre Dame Press.

Gordon, M. (1998). Nursing nomenclature and classification system development. *Online Journal of Issues in Nursing, 3*(2). Available online at http://nursingworld. org/ojin. Accessed October 3, 2008.

Hsieh, H., & Tuite, P. (2006). Prevention of ventilator-associated pneumonia: What nurses can do. *Dimensions of Critical Care Nursing, 25*(5), 205-208.

MacIntyre, A. (1984). *After virtue: A study in moral theory* (2nd ed.). Notre Dame, IN: University of Notre Dame Press.

Olson, E. V. (Ed.). (1967). The hazards of immobility. *American Journal of Nursing, 67* (4), 779-797.

Page, A. (Ed.); Committee on the Work Environment for Nurses and Patient Safety, Institute of Medicine. (2004). *Keeping patients safe: Transforming the work environment of nurses.* Washington, DC: The National Academies Press.

Star, S., & Strauss, A. (1999). Layers of silence, arenas of voice: The ecology of visible and invisible work. *Computer Supported Cooperative Work, 8*(1-2), 9-30.

Steed, C. J. (1999). Common infections acquired in the hospital: The nurse's role in prevention. *Nursing Clinics of North America, 34*(2), 443-461.

8

Practice Breakdown: Interpretation of Authorized Provider Orders

Lisa Emrich ◆ *Kathy Malloch* ◆ *Kathy Scott*

Chapter Outline

SOURCES OF MISINTERPRETATION

The interpretation of provider orders is a critical step in the provision of patient care and has historically been a process that is open to misinterpretation for a variety of reasons. Faulty communication in verbal exchanges between nurses and physicians results in errors ranging from 12% to 91% (Moss, 2005; Proctor et al., 2003; Sutcliffe et al., 2004). Practice breakdown occurs when the orders are missed or misinterpreted and results in instances of carrying out inappropriate orders culminating in an erroneous intervention (Benner et al., 2002). Although illegible handwriting is probably the most common source of misinterpretation, verbal orders not transcribed correctly, verbal orders not understood, incomplete or partial orders, abbreviations, transcription errors, and distractions are also sources of misinterpretation. Missed or mistaken orders are dangerous to patients since essential medications or therapies may be omitted, or wrong therapies or medications may be administered. The incredible volume of communications and frequent interruptions that are present in routine nurse work further contribute to the likelihood of misinterpretation.

Traditionally nurses have been confronted with illegible writing, incomplete orders, and missed orders in the routine transcription of written orders. Verbal orders have long been identified as a source of significant misinterpretation. Both the time lag that occurs between the verbal order and the writing of the order and the significant language dialects and cultural accents of providers have made this practice ineffective and unsafe. Nurses have also been challenged by hierarchical cultures of physician power and control. Challenging physician orders has been frequently discouraged, and if nurses have questioned orders, they have been intimidated or belittled. This dangerous form of power and verbal abuse makes nurses reluctant to further question provider orders. Sometimes nurses are frankly discouraged from calling physicians during night hours. This too is a dangerous practice for patient safety and quality of care that is increasingly being addressed by "rapid response systems" (Devita et al., 2006; Hillman et al., 2005), hospital intensivists who are available during the night hours. Some hospitals (e.g., Stanford University) have identified bullying behavior on the part of any employee as dangerous to a quality of work life and to patient safety, and have instituted required counseling sessions for any employee who is reported more than twice for disruptive or bullying behavior.

DESIGNING FOR SAFETY

The availability of computerized documentation systems and wireless communication technology requires examination of workflow and creation of processes that support appropriate provider orders based on standards of care, accurate interpretation of provider orders by caregivers, and workspace for focus and concentration on safe provision of care.

BENEFITS OF COMPUTERIZATION

The introduction of virtual communication, computerized documentation, computerized physician order entry (CPOE) systems, and monitoring technologies offers processes that can significantly decrease misinterpretation of provider errors and thereby decrease practice breakdown. Computerized provider orders eliminate handwritten orders from practice as well as confusing abbreviations and decimal placements in dosages of medication. Also, the integration of clinical rules, protocols, and alerts within physician order sets become forcing functions that increase the probability of safe, effective patient care interventions. Potential safety benefits from CPOE estimate elimination of 200,000 adverse drug events and savings of $1 billion annually (Hillestad et al., 2005).

The introduction of computers on wheels and handheld personal digital assistants (PDAs) allows caregivers to review orders more quickly, and communicate and clarify orders without leaving the patient's bedside. Multiuser access to the electronic health record and carry-forward logic of historical information decreases time to treatment delays and supports more appropriate patient care. Bates & Gawande (2003) reported that communication failures, particularly those during shift change or "handoffs," may be decreased with this new generation of technology. These systems identify and rapidly communicate problems to clinicians using combinations of cell phones, handheld devices, and paging devices.

TABLE **8.1** **TERCAP**® **Categories of Practice Breakdown**
• Care provider did not follow standard protocol/order
• Care provider missed authorized provider's order
• Care provider carried out unauthorized (not ordered by an authorized provider) intervention
• Care provider misinterpreted telephone or verbal order
• Care provider misinterpreted authorized provider handwriting
• Undetected authorized provider error resulted from the execution of an inappropriate order

As with many practice breakdown categories, missed or misinterpretation of provider orders is often associated with other categories (Table 8.1). Lack of attentiveness or poor clinical reasoning are two categories that can occur before or after the misinterpretation.

POTENTIAL BREAKDOWNS ASSOCIATED WITH COMPUTERIZED PHYSICIAN ORDER ENTRY

It is a truism that no safety measure is foolproof, and each strategy comes with its own potential points of weakness. Computerized Health Care Provider Orders are no exception to this (Han et al., 2005; Koppel et al., 2005; McDonald, 2006).

CASE EXAMPLES/ANALYSES

As discussed previously, practice breakdowns that involve the interpretation of provider orders are commonly associated with other categories of practice breakdown, such as clinical reasoning and attentiveness/surveillance, as the nurse's lack of information or inappropriate application of processes often precedes the misinterpretation of an order. Thus it is relatively rare that an "interpretation of provider orders" would be identified as the primary cause of an error. Because of this, cases that involve nurses' interpretation of provider orders that contribute to practice breakdown have been discussed in other chapters of this book. These cases will be revisited here to discuss specifically the activities associated with the clinical circumstances and nurse activities that pertain to the interpretation of provider orders.

FILLING IN THE BLANKS

In Chapter 4, *Practice Breakdown: Attentiveness/Surveillance*, circumstances were described concerning a patient in long-term care with a confirmed x-ray of fecal impaction. As a result of the x-ray confirmation, the patient's physician provided Ms. Margaret Reyes, a licensed practical nurse, with an order for "Fleet enemas until clear." Nurse Reyes documented the order in the patient's record as "Fleet enemas until clear"; however, the order was transcribed to the patient's medication administration record as "enemas continuously until clear." The transcription to the medication administration record is significantly different from the order that was received and documented. Nurse Reyes questioned the order because she recognized the patient's episode of unresponsiveness following previous administrations of Fleet enemas. She then discussed the order with her nursing supervisor. It is unclear whether the patient's current physician was aware of or did not recall the patient's previous unresponsive episode.

The nurses jointly reconciled their outstanding questions about the order and determined independently that the enemas would be administered every 3 hours until the return was clear. Neither nurse communicated with the physician to discuss their concerns about the patient or attempted to clarify the order until some time later after the patient had received eight Fleet enemas at which time the patient became hypotensive. The nurse then contacted the physician concerning the patient's hypotension at which time the physician ordered intravenous fluids and repeated the order to administer Fleet enemas until the return was clear. At this time the nurse's behavior was appropriate in notifying the physician of the patient's hypotension and requesting clarification of the enema order; however, the nurse did not explain to the physician that the patient had been given a total of eight enemas. In the charge nurse's explanation she stated "I didn't believe it was my responsibility to challenge a physician's order, and I didn't believe I should call my supervisor, the Director of Nursing, in the middle of the night." The physician later noted that he was indeed called in the middle of the night by a nurse who questioned the enema order, but *he* was not informed as to the number of enemas the patient had received. The physician later concluded that the nurse should have used her "common sense and not administered that many [enemas]." There was little evidence that any of the nurses were aware of the dangers of electrolyte and fluid imbalance caused by administering numerous enemas. This is a serious clinical knowledge gap that should have been covered in ongoing care facility education, continuing education, and originally within schools of nursing.

It is important to note the nurse's comment about "challenging" a physician's order and the physician's statement about the nurse not using "common sense." Professionally licensed health care providers give and carry out orders. These actions require their mindful understanding of the patient's current condition and use of this understanding with regard to the actions that are to be taken, the possible complications that could occur as a result of the actions, and the desired outcome of the actions for the benefit of the patient. Because "enemas" were not considered dangerous and/or did not fall into the category of "medication" for these nurses, they apparently felt no need to verify the risks and contraindications for administering multiple enemas. In order for this understanding about the particular vulnerabilities to occur, communication by and between both physicians and nurses is imperative. This is because new information about a patient's circumstance or condition often involves changes that may affect the validity and appropriateness of an existing order. In this case the physician was not informed of the number of enemas administered to the patient. This information would certainly have had a direct impact on the physician's order clarification. However, the physician readily noted that he believed the order he originally provided was indeed appropriate and refused to clarify it further, and later he seemingly chastised the nurse's actions, which could have an intimidating effect on the nurses despite their clear authority to question physician orders. This is especially true for less experienced and less confident individuals who have not developed their sense of "moral agency" (as discussed in Chapter 5) that results in the nurse's reluctance to ask questions in the presence of perceived personal intimidation.

ASSESSING WHAT YOU DO NOT KNOW

Discussion continues in Chapter 5 about a case in which a licensed practical nurse provided care to a patient in a group home. The patient had previously experienced a significant weight loss and was recently diagnosed with an intestinal malabsorption disorder that was treated with surgical placement of a feeding tube. The patient was discharged after a 2-day hospital stay back to the group home. The patient's physician returned the patient to the group home thinking that the staff there was familiar with the patient. This was an environment to which the patient was accustomed and was preferred over admitting the patient to an unfamiliar skilled nursing facility.

The full-time nurse at the group home was a licensed practical nurse, Ms. Mitchell, whose title was "Medical Director." She was not able to secure a tube feeding pump or the feeding solutions for the patient until 4 days after the patient's return to the group home. However, after the pump was received and tube feeding was implemented, it was discovered that the feeding tube was not functioning properly. The patient was subsequently sent to the emergency department where the surgeon revised the feeding tube insertion and again returned the patient to the group home. Although the patient's tube feedings were initiated at that time as ordered, the patient's condition continued to deteriorate. Two weeks later, the patient was transferred to a hospital and died on the day of admission.

The licensed practical nurse stated that she did not worry that it took 4 days to start the ordered tube feedings because the patient continued to drink fluids. Therefore it is clear that Ms. Mitchell did not know the gravity of the patient's malnourished state and the pathologic metabolic effects of the malnutrition. This knowledge deficit resulted in Ms. Mitchell's belief that implementing the tube feedings was not necessarily urgent because the patient was taking fluids by mouth. Ms. Mitchell did not convey the circumstantial delay in initiating the tube feedings to the patient's physician, an action that would be considered important based on the patient's diagnosis and continued weight loss.

The licensed practical nurse stated that she believed since her title was Medical Director, it was her responsibility to make all decisions related to the patient's care, and she was therefore reluctant to contact the consulting registered nurse when concerns were raised. Ms. Mitchell did not recognize that the patient's most immediate need was a satisfactory nutritional intake. Although she contacted the patient's physician concerning the function of the feeding tube, Ms. Mitchell did not recognize and therefore did not convey the patient's continued deterioration to the physician until the time the patient was hospitalized. Although Ms. Mitchell had expressed her reluctance to contact other health care providers, it would also appear that as a licensed practical nurse she had a presumed level of accountability and responsibility that was beyond her professional capabilities. This outcome further supports the need for discharge planning by a team of health care providers to ensure the most appropriate post–hospital care environment that meets the patient's needs.

WHAT DO WORDS MEAN AND TO WHOM?

Chapter 2 discussed a situation in which a registered nurse administered potassium chloride via IV push to a patient. This is a poignant example of miscommunication based on two distinctly different informal interpretations of the word "bolus": a rapid dilute infusion and a rapid infusion of a concentrated potassium chloride solution.

In this situation, Registered Nurse Murphy notified the attending physician of her patient's low serum potassium level in a timely manner. The physician provided Ms. Murphy with an order to give a 40 mEq KCl "bolus." Ms. Murphy repeated, in a conscientious manner, the order word for word back to the physician to verify that she understood the order, which the physician confirmed. Nurse Murphy, indeed, was able to obtain and then administered the KCl bolus. Ms. Murphy's understanding of the word bolus was to rapidly inject medication for purposes of quickly obtaining a desired effect, which is what she did. Although Ms. Murphy, as a registered nurse, is accountable for knowing and/or looking up the potential effects and contraindications of medications that she administers, there is also accountability on the part of the physician to provide clear and concise orders that have clear and concise meanings. In this particular case, the physician's meaning of bolus was somewhat different from Ms. Murphy's meaning of the word.

The kind of practice breakdown presented in this case example is now prevented by the withdrawal of concentrated electrolytes from the immediate availability of the nurse. KCl is also labeled as a "red alert" medication. However, these crucial system redesigns do not resolve the communication breakdown that occurred. This particular concern may only be corrected by using nomenclature that is understood by physicians, nurses, pharmacists, laboratory technicians, respiratory therapists, dieticians, and environmental services in a manner that reduces the number of times the order has to be rewritten or transcribed onto various documents. Breaking down of rigid hierarchies and improving communication are crucial to improving the quality of patient care and patient safety.

SUMMARY

The interpretation of provider orders is carried out frequently on a daily basis by well-meaning health care providers in physicians' offices, patients' homes, acute care facilities, and other health care institutions. Although nurses indeed identify a number of missteps that occur before the error reaches the patient (Page, 2004), nurses who do not question, clarify, or otherwise communicate with the provider of the order place patients at risk for harm by removing any opportunity for the ordering provider to alter his/her decision by being informed of new pertinent patient information. Nurses become very familiar with most treatment and medicinal modalities during the course of their careers and become knowledgeable about many, depending on their practice areas. However, this familiarity and expert knowledge coupled with additional safeguards and resources that are used to enhance nursing practice will further reduce practice breakdowns that occur because of the manner in which a provider order is interpreted. Often the sense of foreboding or unease is a valid sign of a potential error, as is demonstrated in Chapter 1 by Dianne Pestolesi's example of recognizing that the problem of "too many" vials of medication for one dose violates the usual expectation that medication packaging and dosages are *usually* appropriately matched. Staying open and curious as well as fully acknowledging the potential for breakdown is a front-line and effective defense for safety that professionals provide in high-reliability organizations. (Weick & Sutcliff, 2001).

It is the ordering provider's responsibility to communicate his/her medical plan of care for the patient so that nurses and other health care providers understand the primary goals that are desired, and to communicate changes to these goals when they occur. Yet it is the teamwork among health care providers that is essential for the communication of clear and concise orders carried out in a manner appropriate to the clinical area, and in a form that does not lead to misinterpretation. Orders that are vague yet result in the desired goals and outcomes tend to go unnoticed. However, that same vague order may be interpreted in the same or a similar manner and may result in a poor patient outcome. Certainly all health care providers who are involved in a particular patient's care can strengthen their written and verbal communication by using available technology. This will result in an ongoing review of both process and outcomes to optimize patient safety.

References

Bates, D. W., & Gawande, A. A. (2003). Improving safety with information technology. *New England Journal of Medicine, 348*(25), 2526-2534.

Benner, P., Sheets, V., Uris, P., Malloch, K., Schwed, K., & Jamison, D. (2002). Individual, practice, and system causes of errors in nursing: A taxonomy. *Journal of Nursing Administration, 32*(10), 509-523.

Devita, M. A., Bellomo, R., Hillman, K., Kellum, J., Rotondi, A., Teres, D., et al. (2006). Findings of the first consensus conference on medical emergency teams. *Critical Care Medicine, 34*(9), 2463-2478.

Han, Y. Y., Carcillo, J. A., Venkataraman, S. T., Clark, R. S., Watson, R. S., Nguyen, T. C., et al. (2005). Unexpected increased mortality after implementation of a commercially sold computerized physician order entry system. *Pediatrics, 116*(6), 1506-1512.

Hillman, K., Chen, J., Cretikos, M., Bellomo, R., Brown, D., Doig, G., et al. (2005). Introduction of the medical emergency team (MET) system: A cluster-randomised controlled trial. *Lancet, 365*(9477), 2091-2097.

Hillestad, R., Bigelow, J., Bower, A., Girosi, F., Meili, R., Scoville, R., et al. (2005). Can electronic medical record systems transform health care? Potential health benefits, savings, and costs. *Health Affairs, 24*(5), 1103-1117.

Koppel, R., Metlay, J. P., Cohen, A., Abaluck, B., Localio, A. R., Kimmel, S. E., et al. (2005). Role of computerized physician order entry systems in facilitating medication errors. *Journal of the American Medical Association, 293*(10), 1197-1203.

McDonald, C. J. (2006). Computerization can create safety hazards: A bar-coding near miss. *Annals of Internal Medicine, 144*(7), 510-516.

Moss, J. (2005). Technological system solutions to clinical communication error. *Journal of Nursing Administration, 35*(2), 51-53.

Page, A. (Ed.); Committee on the Work Environment for Nurses and Patient Safety, Institute of Medicine. (2004). *Keeping patients safe: Transforming the work environment of nurses.* Washington, DC: The National Academies Press.

Proctor, M. L., Pastore, J., Gerstle, T., & Langer, J. C. (2003). Incidence of medical error and adverse outcomes on a pediatric general surgery service. *Journal of Pediatric Surgery, 38*(9), 1361-1365.

Sutcliffe, K. M., Lewton, E., & Rosenthal, M. M. (2004). Communication failures: An insidious contributor to medical mishaps. *Academic Medicine, 79*(2), 186-194.

Weick, K. E., & Sutcliff, K. M. (2001). *Managing the unexpected: Assuring high performance in an age of complexity.* San Francisco: Jossey-Bass.

9

Practice Breakdown: Professional Responsibility and Patient Advocacy

Patricia Benner ◆ *Kathy Scott* ◆ *Vickie Sheets* ◆
Vicki Goettsche ◆ *Linda Patterson*

Chapter Outline

INTRODUCTION: PROFESSIONALISM AND AGENCY

Professionals are socially constructed agents (Benner, Hooper-Kyriakidis, & Stannard, 1999; Buchanan, 1996) whose justification derives from the benefits they contribute to society that exceed the social costs (Buchanan, 1996). The function of a professional is to serve interests beyond the professional's own self-interest (Hazard, 1996). Professionalism is defined further to include two elements: self-regulation and agency.

SELF-REGULATION

Self-regulation refers to "effective, collective self-regulation by the professional group, including specification of standards of competence for the profession, measures for inculcating in individual members the commitment to these standards, and sanctions for ensuring compliance with them" (Buchanan, 1996, p. 107). (This may also include expulsion from the professional group.) Generally speaking, the question of regulating a professional group's activities arises only where the activity has the potential for seriously affecting the interests of others who are not in a position to protect themselves adequately, such as those involved in a health care professional patient relationship (Buchanan, 1996). The health care profession is much broader than the profession of medicine or physicians and includes many other healing professions, such as nursing, clinical psychology, and pharmacology.

AGENCY

An agent is considered to be one authorized to act or decide on behalf of a principal (Hall, 1996). Agency relations are created because principals recognized that they are incapable of choosing or executing the correct course of action as successfully as were their designated agents, owing to some special expertise of the agent or some disability of the principal. The nurse-patient relationship, like other principal-agent relationships, is characterized by an asymmetry of knowledge and capabilities. The patient as principal is dependent on the nurse as agent because the nurse has knowledge and/or capabilities that he/she lacks. This asymmetry of knowledge or capabilities introduces a risk that the agent would use his or her superior knowledge and ability to pursue his or her own interests or the interests of others at the principal's expense. Therefore some sort of regulation is necessary to provide adequate protection to the principal (Hall, 1996).

NURSE-PATIENT ADVOCACY

Professional responsibility and patient advocacy are central to the nursing role. As noted in the chapters on attentiveness, surveillance, and monitoring, if patient staffing drops too low, nurses will be unable to observe their patients sufficiently to be effective patient advocates. Patient advocacy is the positive, proactive professional stance of a nurse. As a patient advocate, the nurse aligns with the patient to ensure that the patient's concerns are heard and that the patient's well-being is protected. All professionals hold similar social contracts to protect the best interests of their clients/patients, especially when they are unable to adequately protect themselves because of impairment or lack of knowledge. In the judicial system this is called a fiduciary responsibility to the client to ensure that the client's legal rights and best interests are served.

PROFESSIONAL RESPONSIBILITY AND ADVOCACY

Nurse staffing is a situation in which professional responsibility and advocacy are challenged. For example, if a nurse has adequate staffing and support during high demand times (e.g., additional help during a patient crisis on a care unit), he/she has the opportunity to establish the patient's concerns and needs. If this does not occur and he/she does not attend to these patient concerns or well-being, a breakdown in the nurse's social contract of advocating for the patient has occurred.

Another situation involves notification of the provider if the patient's condition changes. A nurse discovers a significant clinical change in the patient's condition, but chooses not to alert the physician in order to follow an informal policy, such as "allow a physician to sleep" or prevent the "physician from being angry about being awakened." In this instance, a serious breakdown has occurred in the nurse's professional responsibility and advocacy.

In one example, a nursing supervisor mandated that no phone calls would be made to physicians during the night. The nurse in charge of caring for a diabetic patient did not overrule this irresponsible and dangerous mandate, and the patient suffered serious harm as a result of a delay in attending to a high blood sugar.

A socially organized practice such as nursing has notions of good internal to the practice (Dunne, 1993; MacIntyre, 1984). By notions of good that are "internal to the practice," MacIntyre means that these notions of what it is good to do are shared and upheld by practitioners—in this case, nurses. Nurses, patients, and their families have a responsibility to protect the vulnerabilities of patients during an illness and hospitalization. If a nurse is dismissive of a patient's concerns about his or her clinical condition, then a breakdown in nursing professional responsibility or advocacy has already occurred. If the nurse is too hurried or too task oriented to notice the patient's and the family's experience, then the level of disclosure on the part of the patient/family will be constrained, and this failed attentiveness will limit the possibility of patient advocacy on the part of the nurse.

As noted earlier, attentiveness (not neglect) and recognition practices (not depersonalization) are notions of good internal to the practice of nursing. They are commonly agreed on and upheld by nurses. A nurse educated to be an excellent nurse can recognize, in most instances, good and poor nursing care, even though it would be impossible to formally list all the precise behaviors and comportments of excellent nursing care.

When nurses recognize substandard care, they carry the professional responsibility to report and/or address substandard care in some manner. For example, in the extremes of the technical worlds of neonatal intensive care units (NICUs), parents, nurses, and physicians struggle with the quality of the environments created for premature neonates. It is never a question of whether an infant can make it on its own.

Astute discernment (*phronesis*) is required to address three major interrelated goals. The first priority in a NICU setting is to meet and assess the particular infant. Discerning the infant's maturity and capacities is crucial since maturation rates vary among infants and are more than just a product of size and intrauterine time. The second goal based on this discernment is to place the infant in a particularized technical/human environment that will support the infant while minimizing technological hazards. The third goal is to foster the social, human birthing of the infant. For example, managing discomfort and pain in these technical environments requires judiciously introducing and teaching human comfort and solace in concert with the infant's ability to tolerate these. Overstimulation can be dangerous. However, social birthing is arrested if the infant does not learn to respond to human touch, comfort, and voice. Introducing these depends on the infant's capacities and readiness. Physiologic demands exist in concert with the demands that the body/social/world relations are adequate for the baby's well-being. Thus the premature infant's survival and flourishing depend on both the human and technical support, just as they do for each full-term newborn infant.

Human beings dwell in human worlds constituted by care, relying on others, and the human *lifeworlds* that they both constitute and are, in turn, constituted by. The knower and the known are intertwined. The intertwining of self and world is so pervasive that it resides in the taken-for-granted background. Often we fail to see and thus forget the concerns that daily suspend us in the webs of care that make up our worlds. Without networks of care or concern, we lack the structures in which to ground our actions and choices. Advocacy is a central moral mandate of excellence in nursing care. Once a particular need for care is recognized, the nurse is responsible for advocating that that care need is met (Benner & Wrobel, 1989).

PROBLEM ENGAGEMENT AND INTERPERSONAL SKILLS

The skills of problem engagement and interpersonal involvement require experiential learning and are essential to effective patient advocacy. For example, clinicians talk about problems of overidentifying with the patient and becoming flooded with feelings in ways that disrupt their perceptual skills. Clinicians must learn skills of involvement that prevent overidentification and emotional flooding over patient problems. However, it is also a problem if the clinician walls off feelings so that the possibilities of attunement are blunted or shut down.

The beginning nurse can feel a generalized anxiety over the demands of learning or the fear of making errors. At this beginning stage, dampening emotional responses can lower anxiety and improve performance. But with the gaining of competency, emotional responses become more differentiated. The practitioner begins to feel comfortable and "at home" in familiar situations and uneasy when the situation is unfamiliar. Learning appropriate emotional responses geared to effective nursing care is central to the formation of character and skills of being a professional nurse or learning *any* professional practice.

When practicing nurses begin to learn differentiated emotional responses that are appropriate to a situation, they can become attuned to the demands and concerns inherent in the clinical situation. They do this through a sense of salience that they have learned experientially as well as through skills of attunement that are specific to the situation. At the competent stage of skill acquisition in nursing, clinical learners can safely pay attention to vague or global emotional responses as a sign that they do not fully understand in the situation because they now recognize a wider array of situations (Benner, Tanner, & Chesla, 2009). At this point, they have a developing sense of *when* they do or do not have a good clinical grasp of the situation.

A sense of salience, tacit memories of similar situations, and skills of attunement are the sources of discovery and early warnings of changes in patients. Emotional responses and communication skills play a key role in perceiving the other's plight and in offering skillful responses. Thus professional responsibility and patient advocacy require prior patient attentiveness and engagement and assertiveness on the nurse's part to make sure that the patient's needs are attended to in a timely manner.

PATIENT AUTONOMY

Much has been written about the importance of patient autonomy in biomedical ethics (Beauchamp & Childress, 2001). However, it is understood that during illness, injury, childhood, or old age, impairments occur that limit the patient's ability to be autonomous. This is yet another reason why the nurse must advocate for patient/family concerns—to augment and support, not usurp, patient autonomy.

Informed consent is one procedure developed to enhance the patient's autonomy. In addition to using formal consent procedures, nurses often coach and teach the patient about the implications and potential outcomes of health care interventions. Informed patient consent is yet another example of the advocacy role of nurses.

Ignoring patients' requests, abandoning patients by leaving the patient care area without notice, or providing substitute care for patients in the nurse's absence constitute breakdowns in professional responsibility. Nurses are responsible for assessing when their patient care assignments are unsafe either because too many patients are assigned to one nurse or because of a patient care assignment for which the nurse has no specific preparation (e.g., use of new technology or equipment without orientation). Likewise, it is inappropriate for a nurse to delegate a medical or nursing responsibility to unlicensed assistive personnel if such an assignment is beyond their safe and/or legal scope of practice. These are difficult areas for nurses employed by institutions that may request or even demand patient care assignments that are unsafe for a particular nurse or even for any nurse to perform alone. In investigating such areas of professional responsibility, it is essential to inquire about the nurse's actions to avoid or to identify whether a patient care assignment is unsafe.

PROFESSIONAL BOUNDARIES

The professional is responsible for delineating and maintaining the boundaries of a therapeutic relationship.

> Professional boundaries are the limits of the professional relationship that allow for a safe, therapeutic connection between the professional and the client. Boundaries protect the space between the professional's power and the client's vulnerability. Establishing boundaries provides a means for professionals to control this power differential and allows for a safe connection based on the client's need (NCSBN, 1996a).

The American Nurses Association (ANA) nursing standards require nurses to maintain "...a therapeutic and professional patient-nurse relationship with appropriate professional role boundaries" (ANA, 2001b, p. 39). These professional boundaries constitute the limits of the ways in which a nurse acts with a patient. They define the best area of behavior for nurses working with patients to meet their needs.

Nurses are professionals, not friends or family members. Boundaries help nurses determine the ways in which they need to behave with patients and to determine what is too much or too little contact. Nurses aim for conduct that is just right.

Professional boundaries established between the provider and the patient assist in identifying the roles and expectations enacted during the nursing therapeutic relationship. When the nurse does not establish boundaries, the therapeutic relationship, which is essential to the delivery of safe and effective care, is compromised. Patients trust that nurses will protect them during a vulnerable time in their lives during illness or injury. This protection is not only limited to preventing medical, nursing, or other errors or advocacy; it extends to the patient's emotional health as well.

Nurses take a holistic approach in providing patient care. This demands that the nurse attend to both the physical and emotional aspects of nursing care. Without the patient's trust, the nurse cannot gain important information regarding the patient's overall health. Nor can the nurse establish the ways in which patients are adapting to the changes in health, coping skills, and relationships with other family and friends that may have an impact on their ability to care for themselves. Ultimately a patient's self-disclosure about the actions they are or are not taking that are affecting their health can be of critical importance in meeting the patient's needs.

It is helpful to visualize a continuum of professional behavior with underinvolvement on one end, overinvolvement on the other, and a center *zone of helpfulness*. Obviously either extreme is undesirable. If nurses are underinvolved with their patients, they will be unable to meet the patients' needs. Overinvolvement presents its own set of problems (discussed below). Any nurse-patient interaction can be plotted on this continuum (Fig. 9.1) (NCSBN, 1996a, pp. 20–21; NCSBN, 1996b).

Conceptualization of this continuum provides a frame of reference for evaluating nurse-patient relationships. Guiding principles for nurse-patient relationships suggest the following:

1. It is the responsibility of the nurse to delineate and maintain boundaries.
2. The nurse works within the zone of helpfulness.
3. The nurse-patient relationship does not become personal.
4. The nurse avoids dual relationships where the nurse assumes an additional role in the life of the patient (e.g., a business relationship).

Under-involved Cold. Distant.	Zone of Helpfulness	Over-involved

FIG. 9.1—Continuum of professional behavior.

5. Post-termination relationships are complex because the patient might need additional services from a facility. It can be difficult to determine when the nurse-patient relationship is really terminated.

The delineation of boundaries may be affected by variables such as the care setting, community influences, patient needs, the nature of therapy, the nursing services provided, the degree of involvement, and patient characteristics. Some patients are more vulnerable because of age, mental status, level of cognitive functioning, and/or past experience. The difference between a caring relationship and an overinvolved relationship can be narrow. A nurse living and working in a remote community will, out of necessity, have business and social interactions with patients.

Establishing appropriate standards is challenging. If the standards are not consistent with real life, they are ineffective and they undermine the authority setting them. In this regard, nurses distinguish between professional and personal interactions. Two types of situations in which boundaries are at risk include boundary crossings and boundary violations.

BOUNDARY CROSSINGS

Boundary crossings may be inadvertent, thoughtless, or even constitute a conscious decision to deviate from an established boundary for a therapeutic purpose. Crossings are brief excursions across boundaries with a return to the established limits of a relationship. Nurses need to be aware of the potential implications of boundary crossings and avoid repeated crossings.

BOUNDARY VIOLATIONS

Boundary violations occur when a nurse violates trust. The therapeutic relationship is damaged when a nurse places his or her own needs before the patient's needs. There are situations where the nurse uses the position of being a nurse to gain access to privileged information, seek opportunity, and use influence over the patient to meet the nurse's need. Boundary violations are a serious type of unprofessional conduct that involves violation of the nurse's fiduciary responsibility to the patient. There is a reversal of roles and secrecy, where the nurse indulges personal privilege leaving the patient caught in a double bind. It is an abuse of the nurse-patient relationship that puts the nurse's needs first instead of assuring the patient that his/her needs are paramount.

Nurses have likes, dislikes, feelings, and attractions. In long-term, sustained relationships that involve intimate and therapeutic activities, nurses cannot help but become close to their patients. Indeed, some have viewed professional boundary violations to be an "occupational hazard" of the caring professions. There are some clues that may or may not be indicative of boundary issues:

1. Self-disclosure—when a nurse discusses personal problems and feelings with a patient.
2. Secretive behavior—when a nurse keeps secrets with the patient or becomes guarded and defensive when interactions are questioned.
3. Selective communications—when a nurse does not report completely or when a patient singles the nurse out repeatedly.

4. *"Supernurse"*—when a nurse believes no one else understands the patient or when a nurse thinks he/she is immune from fostering nontherapeutic relationships.
5. Special treatment by the nurse—when a nurse spends disproportionate amounts of time with a patient or responds differently to an individual patient's requests, trades assignments so the nurse can care for a particular patient, or spends off-duty time with the patient.
6. Special attention to the nurse—when the patient pays special attention to a nurse, waiting up to see him/her, dresses up for the nurse, sends cards or gifts to the nurse, or contacts the nurse after discharge (NCSBN, 1996a, pp. 5-6).

Context is critical when evaluating boundary crossings and boundary violations. The most appropriate stance for the nurses is one of being aware, cognizant of feelings and behavior, and acting in the best interest of the patient. The ANA code summarizes these notions with "the nurse's primary commitment is to the patient" (ANA, 2001a, p. 9).

HISTORICAL CASE STUDY #1: Misplaced Affection, Professional Responsibility

HISTORY

A state mental health facility suspended Ms. Priscilla Rothschild, a registered nurse, pending an investigation into allegations that she had a romantic relationship with a patient. A county recorder indicated that a marriage license named a patient, Mr. Benjamin Huntington, as the groom and Nurse Rothschild as the bride. Nurse Rothschild was permitted to resign from employment, and the situation was reported to the board of nursing.

Nurse Rothschild had worked in general adult psychiatric units throughout her career. She was licensed initially as a licensed practical nurse, then progressed to complete an associate degree in nursing. She obtained her license as a registered nurse in 1995. She had no previous history of employment discipline and no discipline history with the board of nursing.

Nurse Rothschild stated that the relationship with Mr. Huntington consisted of "making popcorn, playing pool, and playing cards." She said she was vulnerable because her common-law husband had deserted her. Mr. Huntington told her that once he got out of the hospital he would be the loving, most wonderful husband she never had. Mr. Huntington reportedly talked her into getting married and convinced her that she could ask the newspaper not to publish the marriage license. Nurse Rothschild reported that she purchased a marriage license for herself and Mr. Huntington.

Nurse Rothschild maintained there was no physical contact between Mr. Huntington and her. She said she knew there was a policy about boundaries, but she was never oriented to it. She had never received any special training for working on the forensics unit even though she had been working there a year.

Nurse Rothschild indicated that she had begun intense psychotherapy and maintained that she was not terminated from her employment, stating, "...I chose to resign." She said she intended to continue her relationship with Mr. Huntington who remained in the facility as a patient. She had sent him care/food packages and indicated that she wanted to visit him at the psychiatric hospital.

The investigation included interviews with other staff members who revealed that Nurse Rothschild had worked for 8 years on the general adult psychiatric unit. She requested transfer to the forensic division after a patient injured her, an incident she attributed to poor staffing. Nurse Rothschild was unable to work for several weeks after her injury and was afraid to return to her previous unit. She thought she would be safer on the forensic unit because it had more staff, including more male staff members working there. The following elements are noted:

1. Nurse Rothschild said she came to understand that having a personal relationship with a patient was wrong and that she didn't understand why she and others engage in personal relationships with patients.

2. Nurse Rothschild became attracted to Mr. Huntington when she observed other staff providing him "incompetent care." She noted that Mr. Huntington had multiple medical problems and that she had a strong medical-surgical background.

3. Mr. Huntington complained constantly of pain, especially migraines. He had filed grievances against staff, and many people lost their jobs.

4. In one instance, Nurse Rothschild discovered that a staff member had removed Mr. Huntington's catheter without deflating the balloon. She began to wonder if his complaints could be valid, and began to advocate for him, but felt the staff was not willing to change because they "did not like him."

5. Nurse Rothschild said she initially denied having a personal relationship with Mr. Huntington because she wanted to protect her mother.

6. Nurse Rothschild was transferred to a women's unit when the marriage license was published.

7. Nurse Rothschild would not make a commitment to her chief nurse that she would not contact Mr. Huntington or allow him to contact her.

8. Nurse Rothschild resigned because she was embarrassed and wanted to continue to see Mr. Huntington.

9. Nurse Rothschild was attracted to Mr. Huntington "because he didn't turn on me." However, Nurse Rothschild had become afraid that Mr. Huntington would "turn on her" and ruin her mother's reputation. She thought Mr. Huntington loved her but that he would "retaliate."

10. Nurse Rothschild continued to visit Mr. Huntington twice a week. She said that the staff approved the continued contact since she was no longer employed there and that she met with his team leader and psychiatrist to assist them by encouraging Mr. Huntington to comply with his treatment plan so he could be discharged eventually.

11. Nurse Rothschild said she had no plans to marry Mr. Huntington but could not terminate the relationship because she was lonely.
12. Nurse Rothschild said that she had never read Mr. Huntington's chart, did not perceive him as having a psychiatric diagnosis, and she was unfamiliar with Axis II diagnosis.

PATIENT'S STATEMENT

1. Mr. Huntington stated that he was romantically involved with Nurse Rothschild but not while she was employed as his nurse.
2. Mr. Huntington indicated that he has no complaints about her and did not believe that she interfered with his therapy.
3. Mr. Huntington wanted to continue the relationship with Nurse Rothschild.

CASE ANALYSIS AND RESOLUTION

Assessment of Care. This situation is characterized as a single, ongoing incident.

Causes. The causes identified in this case are knowledge deficits and errors of judgment.

Awareness. During her interview with the board of nursing, Nurse Rothschild seemed unaware that she had crossed therapeutic boundaries with her patient, and she did not want to end the relationship. Nurse Rothschild said that she left the facility because she was embarrassed. She reported that she was still seeing Mr. Huntington because she feared his retaliation and because she was either unable or unwilling to develop a plan to disengage from the relationship. This was because she said she needed to feel loved.

Responsibility. The responsibility in this case resided in primarily in Nurse Rothschild.

Evidence. Records support and Nurse Rothschild acknowledges having a romantic relationship with a patient.

Outcome/Patient Harm. No harm was assessed in this case.

Remediation Efforts. Nurse Rothschild secured employment at a long-term care facility. She did not plan to return to psychiatric nursing. She was seeing a psychologist because she said, "I want to find out how this could happen to me." Nurse Rothschild characterized herself as having problems setting boundaries, but she said she saw herself as helpless and unable to change.

Legal/Ethical. Nurse Rothschild, indeed, was unable to maintain therapeutic boundaries. However, it remains unclear if she has the knowledge, judgment, and ability to practice forensic psychiatric nursing in the future.

System Issue. In this case, system controls were determined to be lax.

Proposed Resolutions. A stipulation was that Nurse Rothschild participate in the state's Nurse Health Program (NHP).

Violation. The violation in Nurse Rothschild's case was C.R.S. §12-38-117 (1) (f) and (j). It was documented that she:

(f) Has negligently or willfully practiced nursing in a manner which failed to meet generally accepted standards for such nursing practice; and

(j) Had a physical or mental disability which renders her unable to practice nursing with reasonable skill and safety to the patients and which may endanger the health or safety of persons under her care.

Administrative Process. This case was handled through an Alternative Complaint Resolution process. A stipulation and order were agreed on whereby Nurse Rothschild requested and the state board of nursing granted permission to enter the board's confidential impaired professional diversion program in the state.

Action Taken. The following provisions were included in the order:

1. That the state's NHP would report to the board if Nurse Rothschild was terminated from the program for any reason other than successful completion.
2. That if the state's NHP ceases to exist, Nurse Rothschild would be placed on probation with the same requirements as set forth in her state NHP contract.

Disposition. Nurse Rothshild entered the state's NHP and the state board of nursing took no further disciplinary action.

Case Analysis. The registered nurse did not seem to grasp the boundary issue in which she had become involved. She said that since she did not have a physical relationship with the patient while she was employed by the hospital, she did nothing wrong. She had no awareness that she stepped beyond the nurse/client relationship.

The registered nurse showed remorse that the incident reached disciplinary proportions but said she does not regret her relationship with the patient. She said that she had not interfered with the patient's therapy and she intended to pursue the relationship.

The registered nurse perceived herself as a victim, as vulnerable. She did not acknowledge that the patient was being exploited. She did not understand that she was gratifying her personal goals instead of remaining on a professional level, serving the patient's best interests.

The system issues in this case included laxity of procedures that may have promoted boundary problems; it did not seem to be unusual for nurses to socialize with patients/clients.

The system also did not provide this nurse with adequate orientation or education concerning the forensic field of practice and the need to respect boundaries of professional practice. Under the guise of patient advocacy, the nurse became overinvolved with the patient when she thought other staff members were neglecting his care.

System Recommendations. The institution was urged to:

1. Institute policies and procedures to inform and educate staff about expectations regarding the staff-patient relationships.
2. Expect all staff to promote and contribute to an organizational culture in which competence and professional ethics related to professional boundaries are valued and respected.
3. Identify individuals who have had prior boundary issues through staff selection and hiring procedures.

4. Orient and provide ongoing in-service education to address boundary issues.
5. Offer approaches for identifying situations that could lead to boundary issues with an eye to prevention and for dealing with them when they do occur.
6. Practice oversight and supervision to promote early identification and resolution of boundary problems.
7. Review carefully allegations of boundary violations and take appropriate action when warranted.
8. Provide support to staff through counseling, mentoring, discussion groups, and other methods to raise awareness regarding professional boundaries.

References

American Nurses Association. (2001a). *Code of ethics for nurses with interpretive statements*. Washington, DC: ANA.

American Nurses Association. (2001b). *Nursing scope & standards of practice*. Washington, D.C.: ANA.

Beauchamp, T.L., & Childress, J.F. (2001). *Principles of biomedical ethics* (5th ed.). New York: Oxford University Press.

Benner, P., Hooper-Kyriakidis, P., & Stannard, D. (1999). *Clinical wisdom and interventions in critical care*. Philadelphia: W.B. Saunders.

Benner, P., & Wrubel, J. (1989). *The primacy of care: Stress and coping in health and illness*. Menlo Park, CA: Addison-Wesley.

Benner, P., Tanner, C.A., & Chesla, C.A. (2009). *Expertise in nursing practice: Caring clinical judgment and ethics*. New York: Springer.

Buchanan, A. (1996). Is there a medical profession in the house? In R. G. Spece, D. S. Shimm, & A. Buchanan (Eds.), *Conflicts of interest in clinical practice and research* (pp. 105-136). New York: Oxford University Press.

Dunne, J. (1993). *Back to the rough ground: Practical judgment and the lure of technique*. Notre Dame, IN: University of Notre Dame Press.

Hall, M. (1996). Physician rationing and agency cost theory. In R. G. Spece, D. S. Shimm, & A. Buchanan (Eds.), *Conflicts of interest in clinical practice and research* (pp. 228-250). New York: Oxford University Press.

Hazard, G., Jr. (1996). Conflicts of interest in the classic professions. In R. G. Spece, D. S. Shimm, & A. Buchanan (Eds.), *Conflicts of interest in clinical practice and research* (pp. 85-104). New York: Oxford University Press.

MacIntyre, A. (1984). *After virtue: A study in moral theory* (2nd ed.). Notre Dame, IN: University of Notre Dame Press.

National Council of State Boards of Nursing (NCSBN). (1996a). *Quick reference for professional boundaries and sexual misconduct cases: Board of nursing staff*. Chicago: NCSBN.

National Council of State Boards of Nursing (NCSBN). (1996b). *Disciplinary guidelines for managing sexual misconduct cases*. Chicago: NCSBN.

10

Mandatory Reporting

Kathryn Schwed ◆ *Kathy Malloch*

Chapter Outline

How could a nurse as dangerous as Charles Cullen work in 10 hospitals in 16 years—where he says he killed up to 40 patients—and not get caught?" (Under the radar: Secrecy protects bad nurses and doctors. [December 22, 2003], The Record, L-6).

GOALS AND ISSUES IN MANDATORY REPORTING

This chapter focuses on illegal and irresponsible activities that fall outside the boundaries of professional practice. Such illegal actions require reporting the incident to the State Board of Nursing, and the profession is responsible for "policing" such activities, preventing them, and ensuring a due course of legal action when these professional practice boundaries of good practice are crossed. This is where Marx (2001) cautionary notes on a "blame-free" culture are particularly well taken and appropriate. According to Marx (2001), "blame free" can never mean "responsibility free," and some acts fall outside ethical comportment altogether or are egregious and blameworthy. It is one thing to govern and engage in self-improving practices within the bounds of commitment of the practitioners to uphold the standards and notions of good internal to the practice (MacIntyre, 1984), and quite another when practitioners willfully violate the notions of good practice. Some people, within every discipline for whatever reasons, do not choose to uphold the standards of their practice and fall outside ethical practice. Papadkkis (2008), at the University of California San Francisco, found that medical students who had problems with "professional behavior issues" were more likely to be reported to the state board of medicine. This is a cautionary tale for nurse educators as well. Sometimes people may intellectually assent to the standards and boundaries of good practice but

150

not accurately discern in practical situations where these standards are salient and relevant. Others blatantly choose to ignore or violate the professional standards, and therefore do not engage in the essential commitments and formative skills related to good practice. Sometimes, however, extenuating circumstances call for choosing to repair a crisis situation in the only way possible under the circumstances. The patient falling off the operating table had already experienced a serious practice breakdown, and there was no safer choice than to continue the operation under compromised conditions and offer the patient full disclosure of the error. Sometimes in an emergency a contaminated piece of emergency equipment may be used, and when time is essential for saving the patient's life, the safer choice is to use the contaminated instrument to establish the airway or inject an emergency resuscitative medication. Repair of a breakdown situation is the best that can be achieved. Full disclosure to the patient is warranted, and redesign strategies to prevent such future problems are in order. But here we turn to criminal and egregious acts that fall outside of professional practice.

Consider the situation where one nurse observes another nurse reusing a needle. The best practice is to confront the nurse first and inform her that an incident report will be filed with the nursing supervisor. The nurse supervisor, after gathering relevant data about the incident, and consulting with the nurse, will then judge whether it is an isolated and unintended mistake or a repeated pattern of substandard practice. If it is a repeated pattern of substandard practice, the supervisor should report it to the State Board of Nursing. Sometimes nurses over-step the ethical and legal parameters of their practice license. For example, the nurse who administers morphine to a non-responsive, terminally ill patient violates the Nurse Practice Act, and must be reported to the supervisor, and the State Board of Nursing. Accurate documentation of the erroneous medication incident must be completed by the nurse who administered the narcotic. It is the fiduciary and legal responsibility of the nurse to report and attempt to correct practice breakdown of any health care team member including herself.

To address this dilemma, 49 of 59 boards of nursing in the United States have enacted some form of regulatory mandates that require the reporting of certain negative events to their state boards of nursing. The goal of mandatory reporting is to ensure that unsafe practice behaviors are addressed appropriately and in a timely manner. Examples of behaviors in mandatory reporting regulations typically include the following:

1. Suspected theft
2. Physical/verbal abuse, sexual abuse, or exploitation
3. Falsification of documents, cover-ups
4. Repeated medication errors that show a pattern of incompetence or negligence
5. Criminal convictions
6. Patient neglect (such as failing to properly assess, treat, monitor, notify, or intervene)

Unfortunately, the definitions and processes surrounding mandatory reporting vary widely across the country causing confusion and misinterpretation. For example, some states require notification for specific behaviors while others identify general categories of behaviors related to practice breakdown. Some states require that only the "final disciplinary action" be reported concerning any health care professional or voluntary resignation against whom any complaints or reports may have led to disciplinary action. Single incidents of practice breakdown must be reported in some states, while other states require that *patterns* of practice breakdown be reported.

There are advantages and disadvantages to mandatory reporting. The advantage is that negative behaviors are identified and referred to a sanctioned group of professionals familiar with the nurse practice act. One disadvantage is that mandatory reporting often shifts the accountability for the management of practice breakdown from the organization to the regulatory board, thus eliminating the opportunity for early remediation and retraining without the stigma of a state board's involvement. Although the goal of mandatory reporting is to protect the public and ensure prompt resolution of the breakdown, adversarial relationships between nurses, organizations, and boards of nursing and the public may make early detection, local reporting, remediation, and system redesign slower and more contested.

The work of the Practice Breakdown Advisory Panel has been to reconceptualize the nature of error and focus on the creation of a just culture to manage practice breakdown. In a just culture, missteps are viewed as critical learning opportunities for patient safety. The intent is to avoid the tendency to blame individuals for patient safety issues when, in fact, much more may be involved.

Despite mandatory reporting laws, glaring gaps in the system persist. This chapter examines a well-publicized case involving Mr. Charles Cullen, a nurse who is identified by name in the chapter, as his actions received national attention and stories about him appeared in newspapers and other publication outlets in the country. In this regard, the case description is an exception to this book's policy of not revealing a nurse's identity.

In this well-publicized case, the nurse, with seemingly malevolent intent, appeared to have "slipped through the cracks," traveled from one short-term job to another, and escaped detection for many years. The Cullen case is a dramatic example of the failures and opportunities for improvement in the current health care system.

HISTORICAL CASE STUDY #1: The Charles Cullen Case

Mr. Cullen dropped out of high school and enlisted in the Navy soon after his mother was killed in an automobile accident. He first attempted suicide while enlisted, and his behavior reportedly led to a discharge from the Navy in 1984. Mr. Cullen returned to New Jersey and enrolled in a hospital-based nursing program. After graduation, he secured his first nursing position at hospital #1 where he worked first as an employee in its burn unit and subsequently as a "pool" nurse. It was during this period of time that he married and started a family.

Mr. Cullen was not fired from hospital #1 but was forced out when he was given a decreasing number of work assignments for undisclosed reasons. His next position was at hospital #2, in 1992, where he was assigned to work the night shift in the critical care unit. During that time period, he divorced and became infatuated with a female co-worker.

On March 23, 1993, he was arrested for trespassing when he broke into the co-worker's home. He pleaded guilty to downgraded charges and was sentenced to 1 year probation. Also during this period, he attempted suicide for a second time, took 2 months leave from work, and entered psychiatric treatment at a state psychiatric hospital.

Mr. Cullen returned to work as a nurse at hospital #2. During this time, he was questioned about deaths that occurred when he was on duty. On August 30, 1993, Mr. Cullen was caring for Ms. A, a 91-year-old woman in the critical care unit, who was recovering from breast cancer surgery and was showing signs of improvement. On one of the days in the unit, she received a nonprescribed injection of digoxin and died the next day from heart failure. Ms. A's son accused Mr. Cullen of murder. Mr. Cullen underwent and passed a lie detector test, and the accusations ended. Shortly thereafter, Mr. Cullen voluntarily left his job at hospital #2.

Next, Mr. Cullen secured a position at hospital #3 where he became involved in a series of policy infractions. Reportedly he was written up twice: once for tampering with the oxygen settings on the ventilators and once for not following a doctor's orders to discontinue medication. He was fired in August 1997 for "poor performance." After leaving hospital #3, Mr. Cullen crossed over the Delaware River into Pennsylvania and sought work at hospital #4.

Mr. Cullen was described as a loner, angry, and weird by co-workers. He had credit card debts of $40,000 and declared bankruptcy by the time he left hospital #3.

On May 28, 1998, at hospital #4, he was caring for the roommate of Ms. B who received an injection of insulin that seemed to have caused her death. Several nurses were questioned about the sudden death of Ms. B, but nothing conclusive could be determined.

In October 1998, Mr. Cullen was terminated for administering medication at unscheduled times. These infractions were not reported to the board of nursing because, in the view of hospital #4, it did not appear to be the kind of conduct that required reporting.

After leaving his job at hospital #4, Mr. Cullen went to work at hospital #5, which was also located in Pennsylvania. On December 31, 1998, Mr. C received a lethal dose of digoxin on the night Mr. Cullen was caring for him. Mr. Cullen left employment at hospital #5 shortly thereafter and subsequently secured work at hospital #6. He made a third attempt at suicide and was again hospitalized for psychiatric treatment.

Mr. Cullen voluntarily resigned his job at hospital #6 and took a position at hospital #7 in June 2000. He worked in the critical care unit on the night shift. Shortly thereafter, he was accused of leaving unopened boxes of medication containing vials of nitroprusside and procainamide in the sharps container. The boxes were removed, but the very next day there were additional unopened unused vials found in the sharps container. A co-worker reported him to the hospital administrator. When questioned, Mr. Cullen was unable to explain why he was storing medication that was not seen as addictive and had little street value. The hospital administrator terminated Mr. Cullen and reported him to the Pennsylvania Board of Nursing, which took no formal action against him.

His next place of employment was at hospital #8 in Pennsylvania. He was fired after 16 days of employment. The documented reason was because he was unable to get along with his co-workers.

Mr. Cullen then crossed back over the river into New Jersey and took a job at hospital #9. The hospital's check of his credentials and past employment history revealed that he had valid nursing licenses in New Jersey and Pennsylvania. No derogatory information was relayed by any past employer to hospital #9 since employment policies at most of these facilities allowed only for the confirmation of his dates of employment. Mr. Cullen's past employment history was not revealed.

While at hospital #9, Mr. Cullen was assigned to work on the night shift in the critical care unit. In June 2003 he cared for Mr. D, a patient diagnosed with cancer. Mr. D suffered sudden heart failure after being injected with a nonprescribed dose of digoxin. Prior to this incident, two other patients had suffered life-threatening decreases in blood sugar caused by insulin overdoses. The hospital did not report the incidents to the police or to the New Jersey Board of Nursing at that time, but they did consult with a doctor from the New Jersey Poison Information and Education System.

Mr. Cullen continued to work at hospital #9. On July 27, 2003, Mr. E, who was in the ICU at the hospital, received a nonprescribed dose of digoxin and died of heart failure the next morning. The lab results showed toxic levels of digoxin in the patient's system.

Meanwhile, the hospital received feedback from the expert at the New Jersey Poison Information and Education System. He informed hospital authorities that he intended to report the matter to the New Jersey Department of Health and Senior Services. Eight days later, Mr. F, another patient, suffered a precipitous drop in his blood sugar and died. The hospital administrator immediately notified the county prosecutor's office and that office launched an investigation.

The prosecutor's office reviewed pertinent medical records and on December 8, 2003, alerted the New Jersey Board of Nursing of an impending arrest. On December 12, 2003, Mr. Cullen was arrested and charged with one count of murder and one count of attempted murder.* On request made by the New Jersey Board of Nursing that very day, Mr. Cullen signed an interim order of voluntary surrender pending the completion of the criminal case. On April 29, 2004, after Mr. Cullen pleaded guilty to multiple counts of murder and

---

*Ultimately, Mr. Cullen pleaded guilty to causing the deaths of 29 patients and was sentenced to life imprisonment in New Jersey and Pennsylvania. (See N.J.S.A. 26:2H-12.2 N.J.S.A. 45:1-28 et seq. N.J.S.A. 45:1-33 et seq N.J.A.C. 13:37-5.8, 5.9) (New Jersey State Attorney's Office, Public Files.)

attempted murder in County Superior Court, he signed a consent order with the New Jersey Board of Nursing agreeing to permanently surrender his license to be deemed a license revocation. His license was also revoked in Pennsylvania.

ANALYSIS

This registered nurse's story has had a devastating impact on its victims, their families, the public, and the nursing community.

But it has also focused attention on reforms needed to improve the health care system. While patterns of errors and acts of professional misconduct are supposed to be reported under most reporting regulations, the Cullen case underscores the ways in which a single error or act can be dubbed as *simple negligence* when it may be indicative of a more extensive pattern of error and misconduct.

COLLABORATION

The case emphasizes the importance of open and honest communication between various interested individuals/entities, that is, the lines of communication between past and current employers, between staffing agencies and facilities where a nurse is assigned to work, between-state agencies (e.g., professional licensing boards, departments of health, and local police or prosecutors), and between sister state boards of nursing. These communications are all vital in developing a comprehensive system where information is passed along to individuals or entities that have a need to know about a particular nurse.

CONFIDENTIALITY

The person or reporting entity needs to keep the issues confidential at all stages since it can be detrimental to the investigation to discuss the issues with others and with the subject himself or herself, and may cause a serious breach of the subject's right to a fair and confidential hearing. Confidentiality is intended to protect licensees who have been exonerated after investigation. Clearly, a licensee who has not been found to have engaged in actionable misconduct should not have to worry about losing a job or not getting a job because an employer learns that he/she has been the subject of a prior investigation.

MOTIVATION FOR REPORTING

Preventing professional practice breakdown and intentional misconduct is a commonly held and serious responsibility of every professional. It is important that the person filing a report act in good faith without ulterior motives. The motivation to report does not presuppose patient harm; it may be stimulated by a concern for the potential harm that certain conduct may pose. Co-workers and supervisors who work day in and day out with a licensee need to know about their colleagues' histories because they are in the best position to know when there are early signals of distress. Without accusatory or punitive intent, they need to look for these behavioral signals, which are often a precursor to practice breakdown or intentional misconduct.

PREMATURE REPORTING

Reporting suspicions about poor practice is avoided because it is oftentimes too subjective, especially where a nurse may have personality conflicts or eccentricities that may be at the heart of an allegation. More than mere suspicion is necessary for a report to go forward; a tangible documented incident or error is needed. However, professional colleagues carry a professional responsibility to discuss directly any concerns about care practices that might fall below standards of care or endanger patients. False reporting on mere suspicion is dangerous and is to be avoided. Yet in a fast-paced practice such as nursing, practitioners are expected to cross monitor and support good practice of colleagues without an accusatory or punitive spirit. This kind of local team support is expected of all professional practice environments as a central step in ongoing practice improvement.

COOPERATION

All persons or entities need to cooperate with a board of nursing investigation and provide information and documentation as needed. One of the problems in tracking the pattern of errors attributable to Mr. Cullen was the fact that some of his previous employers did not appear to have fully documented the precise reasons for his termination or forced resignation. All infractions and errors need to be fully documented. However, reports to a board of nursing are not taken at face value. Board staff members undergo major efforts to validate information and to examine all sides of an issue. Substantial board inquiries and investigations take place before any decision is made or before it can even be determined if there are grounds for disciplinary action. The purpose of this validation process is to eliminate those reports that are clearly without merit or do not rise to the level of conduct that would warrant licensing intervention. Sometimes a report will document initially one issue only to find that the investigation discloses other issues or parties involved leading to examination of additional incidents or conduct to be examined.

CONDUCTING ROUTINE CRIMINAL BACKGROUND CHECKS

Conducting routine criminal background checks constitutes positive reform. Initial criminal background checks and corresponding flagging systems are being used in which an employer or board is notified if there is a new arrest or conviction. Increasingly more employers and state boards of nursing are using these approaches as one means for screening applicants for a job or a license. Formerly, it was common practice for a state board of nursing or employer to simply ask a question about an applicant's criminal history and presume that they were getting a truthful answer. More recently, verification of the answers is accomplished through an objective review of an applicant's possible criminal background. In this case, the registered nurse responded truthfully to the question on his license application in New Jersey because his arrest for trespassing did not occur until years after he completed his application. At that time, no flagging system was in place to alert the board of nursing that the arrest had occurred.

INCREASED VIGILANCE IN HIRING AND LICENSING PRACTICES

Employers and state boards of nursing clearly need to know when a nurse has been terminated or permitted to resign in lieu of termination when the reason is related to substandard patient care or intentional abuse. This is especially true when the nurse lives in a border state where crossing over a river or state line is commonplace. Close scrutiny needs to be paid whenever a licensee has an employment history with a series of short-term positions, large gaps in time, or unexplained absences. Short-term assignments and gaps in employment may simply be the product of choice and represent a licensee's need for flexibility and work variety. But it can also be cause for suspicion. As in the Cullen case, it may be indicative of sinister motivations, such as the inability to hold on to a job for longer than 6 months or a purposeful desire to remain unnoticed.

Asking probing questions about a licensee's past employment history is also a means to detect a problematic work record. Licensees who take per diem assignments from nurse registries can be quizzed about whether they have been placed on an ineligibility list. While sometimes these *Do Not Use* lists are used to weed out personality conflicts, they are just as often used to avoid using a licensee who has been the subject of repeated error.

Oftentimes the employment application is not filled out completely, especially when dates of employment are fudged to account for all time gaps. It is up to an astute interviewer to observe these gaps and make appropriate inquiries where necessary.

Hospitals have been traditionally reluctant to reveal detailed work histories about past employees, even when they have been terminated for cause. They are much more inclined to simply verify the dates of employment and provide no substantive evaluation of work performance. However, this is beginning to change. For instance, the Cullen case has spurred reform in New Jersey, where a law was recently passed to provide civil immunity to hospitals that reveal information about practice breakdown as long as the report is made in good faith, without malice, and on the request of another hospital. It remains to be seen how the law will be implemented, but it was designed to help.

"RED FLAGS"

Pyrek (2003) identified 13 *red flags* that require attention and investigation. The list includes the following:
1. The nurse is uncommonly accurate in predicting patient's demise.
2. A higher percentage of deaths occur while the nurse is on duty.

3. Patient deaths are unexpected by staff or family, and the patient dies alone.
4. Co-workers often report allegations to investigators.
5. Witnesses report seeing the nurse with the patient shortly before the patient unexpectedly died.
6. Death is caused by substances that are readily available, not easily detectable, and not routinely checked at autopsy, including insulin, digoxin, lidocaine, epinephrine, and other respiratory-paralyzing agents. Syringes, IV lines, and feeding tubes are likely portals of entry.
7. If a code is called, ECG strips are often not placed in the chart.
8. The nurse has difficulty with personal relationships.
9. Prior employment records show questionable incidents.
10. The nurse is given nicknames by the staff before a concern is reported.
11. The nurse insists patient(s) died of natural causes.
12. The nurse fails to show remorse for victims and justifies his/her actions.
13. Other patients or families complain about the nurse, but their comments are often ignored.

SUMMARY

The horribly egregious nature of a serial killer cannot be overestimated. There are, however, several strategies and actions that nurses can take to identify potential sources of concern that may result in untoward outcomes or death. It is essential that nurses listen carefully to patients or families who complain that, in their view, a health care provider intentionally harmed them. Regardless of these assertions, members of the health care team need to track and investigate them, and if found wanting, report them to legal authorities and licensing boards. Employers should not allow suspected individuals to resign in lieu of termination or an investigation into wrongdoing. Finally, nurses and other health care team members must be knowledgeable and educate others to recognize red flags, as this responsibility rests with all members of the healthcare system.

References

Bowman, B. (2004, January 16). Another lie in nurse's past. *Courier News.*

Campbell, C., & Patterson, M. J. (2004, March 14). Code of silence gives rogue nurses a dangerous past. *Star-Ledger, 1,* 20-21.

Hader, R. (2005). How do you measure workforce integrity? *Nursing Management, 36* (9), 32-36.

MacIntyre, A. (1984). *After virtue* (2nd ed.). Notre Dame, IN: University of Notre Dame Press.

Marx, D. (2001). *Patient safety and the "just culture": A primer for health care executives.* New York: Columbia University Press.

Papadakis, M.A., Arnold, G.K., Bland, L.L., Holmboe, E.S., Lipner, R. (2008). Performance during internal medicine residency training and subsequent disciplinary action by state licensing boards. *Archives of Internal Medicine 148*(11), 869-876.

Perez-Pena, R., Kociekiewski, D., & George, J. (2004, February 29). Through gaps in system, nurse left trail of grief. *The New York Times, 1*, 32-33.

Perez-Pena, R., Kociekiewski, D., & Peterson, M. J. (2003, December 17). Hospitals didn't share records of nurse suspected in killings. *The New York Times, 1*, B8.

Pyrek, K. M. (2003). Healthcare serial killer: Recognizing the red flags. *Forensic Nurse.* Available online at http://www.forensicnursemag.com/articles/391feat1.html. Accessed October 6, 2008.

System failed patient four ways. (2004, November 21). *Star-Ledger*, p. 1, 14.

Under the radar: Secrecy protects bad nurses and doctors. (2003, December 22). *The Record*, L-6.

11

Organizational Use of TERCAP®: Shifting From a Quality Management to a Whole-Systems Approach

Kathy Scott

Chapter Outline

Serious quality problems continue to exist in the health care industry in spite of a highly trained workforce of skilled and motivated people who are technically proficient (Chassin & Galvin, 1998). A fundamental shift in thinking is required to create safe and reliable practice environments for technically proficient practitioners. This shift begins with the recognition that a quality management approach is not enough, and that a whole-systems management approach is required.

QUALITY MANAGEMENT VERSUS A WHOLE-SYSTEMS MANAGEMENT APPROACH

Quality management operates within an existing paradigm that can be learned and applied as an independent set of tools and methods. It is an approach in which care providers analyze the elements or parts of a problem or situation to gain a better understanding of it. Alternately, a systems approach considers learning through an understanding of the whole—the parts themselves *and* the interaction of the parts. Moving forward with the Institute of Medicine (IOM) recommendations related to error prevention in health care will require a whole-systems approach. That is an approach that seeks to understand the

160

parts and their interactions as well as the broader context in which they are embedded, including the expectations, assumptions, habits, behaviors, history, and traditions that influenced a situation. A better understanding of the whole is a prerequisite for intelligent leadership and reliable results in today's health care organizations.

SENTINEL EVENTS AND THE PATIENT SAFETY MOVEMENT

Sentinel events are any unexpected occurrence involving death or serious physical or psychological injury, or the risk thereof. The phrase *or the risk thereof* includes any process variation for which a recurrence would carry a significant chance of a serious, adverse outcome. The events are called *sentinel* because they signal the need for immediate investigation and response (Speelman, 2001). In 1998, The Joint Commission on the Accreditation of Healthcare Organizations implemented standards and recommendations related to identifying, reporting, analyzing, and presenting sentinel events that had become more commonly reported in health care organizations throughout the country. These recommendations, however, fell short of expectations, and these unfulfilled expectations provided a segue to the patient safety movement.

The patient safety movement, while clearly visible, is still in its infancy. Many hospitals continue to punish care providers for the errors they make, and regulatory bodies are seen as searching for villains and punishing those who get caught. Meanwhile, the focus of many health care leaders has been on acquisitions, mergers, reimbursement, and revenue, rather than on the core focus of patient care. The patient safety movement will not progress until health care leaders move away from traditional models of management that focus almost exclusively on the bottom line to a multidimensional approach that focuses on other dimensions of organizational fitness—that is, the normative, strategic, and operational aspects of the organization (Schwaninger, 2000).

ORGANIZATIONAL USE OF TERCAP®

The Practice Breakdown Advisory Panel (PBAP) developed and used the Taxonomy of Error, Root Cause Analysis and Practice Responsibility (TERCAP) audit (introduced in Chapter 1) as one method in a study of practice breakdown in multiple health care settings. The goal of this research (Scott, 2004) was to study selected error-events and identify the multiple individual, team, system, and cultural contributors to the practice breakdown that resulted in harm to a patient. It was asserted that an enhanced analysis would result within the context of a comprehensive framework by incorporating TERCAP into the root cause analysis and investigative process. Data collection included systematic root cause analysis findings and data obtained from medical records, staffing schedules, and physician and employee interviews. TERCAP proved to be a very useful data collection instrument for organizing and analyzing the data.

The purpose of this chapter is to examine the findings from one typical error-event that occurred in a hospital setting. The failure of this event was that a post-surgical patient's care was inadequately monitored, and this failure resulted in significant harm to the patient. Not surprisingly, findings revealed that harmful patient care errors resulted from multiple failures by many people working in complex systems while carrying out routines of daily practice.

The researcher collected specific information about an error-event that included data from the root cause analysis process and from interviews with individuals who were directly and indirectly involved. The error-event is described in detail to assist readers in gaining a comprehensive multifaceted overview of the case through a whole-systems approach that is rich with information and carries implications for professional education and training, system design, and cultural transformation.

HISTORICAL CASE STUDY #1: Failure to Adequately Monitor a Postsurgical Patient

DESCRIPTION OF THE EVENT

This error-event involved inadequate monitoring of a patient who had undergone an elective surgical procedure. A certified nursing assistant made a proximal error when she failed repeatedly to report abnormal vital signs to a registered nurse assigned to the patient. The patient was receiving narcotics via a patient-controlled infusion device. The patient was obese and had a large neck. He also had a history of sleep apnea. This combination of factors may have combined to cause respiratory depression that resulted in abnormal vital signs.

The nursing assistant's reporting was inadequate, and consequently the registered nurse was unaware of the patient's low blood pressure. The patient's condition subsequently deteriorated to the point where he was seriously compromised and near death, and may have been permanently harmed as a result.

DEMOGRAPHICS

This error-event occurred in a community hospital setting. In this event the investigation revealed that three people made errors that constituted unsafe acts and resulted in harm to the patient. These included the nursing assistant, the registered nurse (who was prepared at the associate degree level), the registered nurse in the charge/staff nurse role, and a board-certified surgeon.

The registered nurse and surgeon agreed to be interviewed, but the nursing assistant declined. Three additional people were indirectly involved and participated in the interview process. They were the oncoming registered nurse (prepared at the associate degree level of nursing), a registered (associate degree) respiratory therapist on duty, and the associate degree registered nurse house supervisor.

The root cause analysis group included two of the people who engaged in unsafe acts, one other person who was directly involved, and six additional people with expertise in the routine practices and processes of the surgical unit and related areas.

SETTING ELEMENTS

The incident occurred during one 12-hour shift between Friday at 7:00 PM and Saturday at 7:30 AM. All of the individuals directly involved in the event were working a regularly scheduled shift. The two employees who carried out the unsafe acts were working the night shift. The surgeon involved in the case had not worked the night before.

BACKGROUND INFORMATION

In the hospital setting, patients often receive pain medication through a pump that provides a specific dose on demand with a programmed maximum dose allotment. The patient-controlled analgesia (PCA) pump is programmed to deliver specific, small dosages of the medication only when the patient pushes a specified button. Therefore, if the patient is unable to push the button, he/she does not receive any more of the medication via the pump.

NARRATIVE OF THE EVENT

A young man, Mr. Steve Goldberg, was admitted to a surgical unit at 6:00 PM after an elective laparoscopic gastric bypass surgical procedure. Mr. Goldberg was stable at the time of admission and was receiving a patient-controlled narcotic infusion at a "high-normal" range for pain management via a PCA pump. He was receiving oxygen via a nasal cannula at 2 liters per minute.

On admission to the surgical unit, Mr. Goldberg's blood pressure was stable at 142/87. He stated that he was comfortable but at times appeared uncomfortable and restless. At 8:50 PM, the patient denied having pain and wanted his oxygen removed. His oxygen levels were adequate, and the respiratory therapist removed the oxygen cannula at that time but left it in the room per routine procedure. Mr. Goldberg continued to be restless throughout the evening and was observed repositioning himself in the bed for comfort.

At midnight, the nursing assistant, Ms. Veronica Martin, removed the blood pressure cuff from Mr. Goldberg's arm for comfort after recording a blood pressure of 92/44. She did not inform the registered nurse, Ms. Margaret Bennington, of the decrease in blood pressure but recorded the blood pressure on her worksheet, a nonpermanent record on a clipboard that contained the vital signs of the patients assigned to her. The nursing assistants used the worksheet to record vital signs for the registered nurse's review before documenting them in the permanent medical record.

At midnight, however, Nurse Bennington was busy admitting a new patient. One hour later (1:00 AM), Nursing Assistant Martin repeated the blood pressure measurement and documented a blood pressure of 76/34 on her worksheet.

Again, Nursing Assistant Martin did not report the increasingly lowered blood pressure to Nurse Bennington.

Nurse Bennington stated that at 2:45 AM she checked on Mr. Goldberg and characterized him as being restless, able to hold a conversation, and complaining of being too hot. Nurse Bennington gave Mr. Goldberg a cool wet cloth and took his blanket off. Nurse Bennington did not check any additional vital signs or ask to see the recorded blood pressure readings, stating that she assumed the patient was stable.

One hour later (3:45 AM), Nursing Assistant Martin was assigned for a short time to another unit. She did not communicate any information to Nurse Bennington regarding Mr. Goldberg before leaving the unit. She returned approximately one and one-half hours later.

At 5:15 AM, Nursing Assistant Martin returned to the clinical unit and recorded Mr. Goldberg's vital signs as 77/34, pulse 100, and respirations 20. Nursing Assistant Martin gave Nurse Bennington a brief report on a second patient and then left to take a third patient's vital signs.

At 5:30 AM, the surgeon, Dr. Steel, came in earlier than his usual time to evaluate the patient. Dr. Steel's intentions were to quickly assess the patient and then leave for the airport where he had an early commercial flight to catch. Dr. Steel stated that he could hear Mr. Goldberg snoring as he approached the room, and when he entered Mr. Goldberg's room, he found the patient cyanotic from the neck up and unresponsive to verbal stimuli. Dr. Steel left the room to get Nurse Bennington for help, and together they returned to Mr. Goldberg's room.

Nurse Bennington stated that Mr. Goldberg was positioned on his side, which was unusual, and that it was obvious he wasn't doing well. His color was poor, respirations were slow, and he was unresponsive. At this time, Nurse Bennington repositioned Mr. Goldberg on his back to open his airway and improve his breathing.

Over the next 50 minutes, the narcotic infusion was discarded and Mr. Goldberg received two doses of medication to reverse the effects of the narcotic infusion. His arterial blood gases were assessed, and his oxygen was reinstituted via nasal cannula. He remained on the surgical unit for approximately 50 minutes while, according to each of the three staff members interviewed, Dr. Steel was reclined in a chair in the corner of the patient's room or at the nurses' station making phone calls while they suggested interventions to him.

The three registered nurses interviewed expressed concerns about their perceived delays in treatment after Mr. Goldberg was discovered in his unstable condition, and attributed the delays to waiting for Dr. Steel to take the initiative. According to Dr. Steel, he reinstituted Mr. Goldberg's oxygen, instructed Nurse Bennington to turn off the patient-controlled narcotic infusion, and to give the medication to reverse the effects of the narcotic.

Dr. Steel left to catch his plane before the patient was stabilized. Mr. Goldberg showed some improvement before Dr. Steel left. Dr. Steel stated that he thought the patient's systolic blood pressure was approximately 100, and he had oxygen saturation levels of approximately 92%. Neurologically, his pupils were reacting slightly; he was posturing on his left side and flaccid on the right side, and remained unresponsive to verbal stimuli.

Mr. Goldberg was transferred to the intensive care unit at 6:20 AM where the nurses in the ICU quickly increased the oxygen support and added intravenous vasopressors per protocol after consultation with the on-call physician in internal medicine, Dr. Asvall. A gap of approximately 30 minutes occurred between the time Dr. Steel left for the airport and the time Dr. Asvall arrived to manage the case.

PATIENT OUTCOME

A near-death event and possible permanent patient harm was attributed to a series of unsafe acts. The unsafe acts resulted in respiratory and circulatory compromise, brain ischemia, and a small myocardial infarction (heart attack) to a young man, Mr. Steve Goldberg, who had undergone elective surgery.

THE PRIMARY CATEGORY OF ERROR

The primary category of error in this event is inappropriate judgment by Nursing Assistant Martin, the individual most proximal to the patient's harm. Nursing Assistant Martin's actions demonstrated inappropriate judgment in not notifying Nurse Bennington of Mr. Goldberg's condition at the time she obtained a blood pressure reading that was substantially lower than the patient's prior recorded blood pressures.

INDIVIDUAL CONTRIBUTIONS

It is difficult to know why Nursing Assistant Martin did not report her findings to Nurse Bennington because Nursing Assistant Martin did not participate in the interview or RCA process. She had the experience and training to know that the change in blood pressure was significant and reportable. Members of a review team that conducted root cause analyses wondered if Nursing Assistant Martin thought the blood pressure reading was inaccurate because of equipment problems. Mr. Goldberg was obese, a condition that can make accurate blood pressure readings from an arm cuff difficult and inaccurate, even when a large-sized cuff is used. Regardless, the appropriate action and standard operating procedure in the unit was for a nursing assistant to inform the registered nurse so that the registered nurse could then evaluate the patient and determine the underlying problem.

Nursing Assistant Martin did not seek assistance from Nurse Bennington immediately or over the course of the next several hours in spite of additional blood pressure readings that were well below the norm for any healthy adult. As a result, Mr. Goldberg's deteriorating status was not noticed and he was harmed.

In addition to inappropriate judgment, Nursing Assistant Martin's actions also reflect a *communication failure* with Nurse Bennington, verbally and in writing. Not only did Nursing Assistant Martin fail to seek out a face-to-face interaction with Nurse Bennington, Nursing Assistant Martin did not initiate any actions through her documentation to ensure that Nurse Bennington reviewed Mr. Goldberg's vital signs.

Nursing Assistant Martin's actions also demonstrated a *lack of attentiveness or surveillance* of Mr. Goldberg. She did not return and take additional blood pressure readings or attempt to replace any equipment as a result of the low blood pressure readings. Rather, she maintained her routine schedule, added no further interventions, and resumed her routine rounds to collect vital sign readings. Nursing Assistant Martin knew that she would be reassigned to another unit at some time during the shift. Perhaps this knowledge was distracting to her and contributed to her lack of attentiveness.

Nurse Bennington demonstrated *poor judgment* when she did not adequately supervise an unlicensed assistive person, Nursing Assistant Martin. It is the responsibility of the registered nurse assigned to a specific patient (in this case the staff/charge registered nurse) to oversee a patient's care whether or not components of that care are delegated to a certified nursing assistant or to another team member. This supervisory oversight was not present in this error-event, and this left a "fresh" postoperative patient who required monitoring and more frequent assessment per nursing standards without registered nurse oversight.

A registered nurse has the authority and responsibility to assess, evaluate, and use nursing judgment when caring for patients during times that unlicensed assistive personnel are assisting with, but not replacing, the functions the registered nurse is expected to carry out (NCSBN, 1995). The staff/charge registered nurse, Nurse Bennington, did not act responsibly to meet the needs of Mr. Goldberg, a postsurgical patient, and used *inappropriate judgment* when she focused on specific tasks or demands and did not recognize the vulnerabilities of a patient that, in this instance, involved the potential for a compromised airway secondary to his anatomy and narcotic dosing.

Nurse Bennington's actions or inactions also demonstrated a *lack of attentiveness or surveillance* related to Mr. Goldberg's compromised respiratory and hemodynamic status, and related to symptoms that went undetected for several hours, according to the arterial blood gas results. Further, Nurse Bennington did not effectively monitor Mr. Goldberg, a postoperative patient, during an unsafe period of time and did not detect substandard care on the part of Nursing Assistant Martin.

Nurse Bennington also used *inappropriate judgment* in that she did not insist on having adequate information on a postoperative patient. She did not seek out Mr. Goldberg's information and therefore was unable to evaluate, in a timely manner, Mr. Goldberg's response to therapy such as narcotic infusion and pain management. In addition, she did not demonstrate good judgment in supervising Nursing Assistant Martin, a person she described as "a little too independent" and "very task oriented," and as someone who did not pass along information "unless asked." Knowing this, Nurse Bennington could have given Nursing Assistant Martin more specific instructions and sought out the information Nurse Bennington needed to adequately monitor the patient. Nursing Assistant Martin was inadequately monitored and Nurse Bennington did not evaluate the effectiveness of the delegated assignment.

TEAM CONTRIBUTIONS

This situation involved poor communication, coordination of effort, and follow-up that occurred between Nurse Bennington, the staff/charge registered nurse, and Nursing Assistant Martin. The team contributed to the delay in responding to a deteriorating patient through *lack of or poor communication, coordination of effort, follow-up, feedback, and competency.*

Nurse Bennington, the staff/charge registered nurse, expressed reluctance to overload the other registered nurse with whom she was working. Her concern for his competency affected the coordination of care on the unit. Nurse Bennington stated that the novice registered nurse had recently completed his orientation and described him as "smart, but lacks life experience." Thus, because of this reluctance to overload her team member, Nurse Bennington took the midnight patient admission assignment, which would normally have been assigned to the other registered nurse. With this additional patient, she now had five patients of the nine on the unit with the help of Nursing Assistant Martin, who was assigned to all nine patients. This was considered a "reasonable" assignment in this particular unit where the team often assumed the care for seven patients per one registered nurse, depending on patient acuity. Normally the two registered nurses would assist each other as needed throughout the shift. The inexperienced registered nurse reportedly did not assist Nurse Bennington with her workload, however, because "he had his hands full" according to Nurse Bennington.

A team dynamic that repeatedly surfaced in the interviews was the "paralysis" of the team in *communicating with each other and coordinating the care* for the patient's deteriorated condition because of the presence and behavior of the surgeon, Dr. Steel. The participants in the meeting reported that the surgeon's actions and inaction contributed to the delays in patient interventions at a time when fast action was needed. One registered nurse stated that, in hindsight; she would "go after it a little bit more aggressively next time. I wished after it was over that I had, regardless of the doctor." She added, "But a doctor that is sitting back in a chair looking over stuff and asking the same question over and over again—I don't remember what it was but he asked the same question three times that had nothing to do with what was going on."

Dr. Steel also contributed to poor communication, coordination of effort, and follow-up by leaving, or perhaps abandoning, a patient for whom he had responsibility; this resulted in a 20- to 30-minute gap in physician coverage at a time when the patient was unstable.

In nursing practice, patient abandonment occurs when a nurse accepts an assignment and responsibility for patients yet leaves the assignment without notifying his/her supervisor or other responsible staff member and does not communicate the need for another nurse to cover a patient's condition and needs (Benner et al., 2002).

Abandonment is not as clearly defined for physicians in a hospital setting. In this case, however, Dr. Steel removed himself from a newly unresponsive and unstable patient before obtaining replacement coverage, although he may have been available by phone during the gap.

Dr. Steel and the team also failed to communicate effectively with each other about the patient's care needs. One registered nurse stated the following related to Dr. Steel:

> "I felt like he was much disengaged. He was in his own thought process. He was concerned about his flight. I didn't know what his thought processes were. If he could have shared what he was thinking or what his plan was, or shared *anything*, it would have felt better because then we could have had a dialogue. But there was no dialogue."

Dr. Steel's perception of the situation was quite different from the rest of the group, however. He stated that he felt that he "actually came out the hero in the deal" in that he happened to be "the lucky one that found Mr. Goldberg." "From that point of view" he noted, "I feel good that I was there and intervened."

The communication within the group was such that Dr. Steel did not receive any *feedback* of the group's perception of his actions nor did he learn of their concerns about his decision to leave the patient. The gap also included the house supervisor registered nurse who was the person on the team with the authority to take action.

SYSTEM CONTRIBUTIONS

Two system factors contributed to the error-event. The first was a lack of adequate system controls, or standard operating procedures and training, for the following two critical operations. The first was caring for the high-risk surgical patient and reporting of critical data between registered nurses and nursing assistants. The second was lack of follow-up for a critical operation—physician coverage for high-risk patients.

The surgical unit did not have adequate system controls. Each registered nurse had his/her own particular way of obtaining information from the nursing assistants rather than following a standardized process. This may have contributed to the error in this instance if the nursing assistant's expectations were for the registered nurse to review the worksheet and vital signs on a regular basis without the nursing assistant assuming responsibility for initiating the activity.

Poor system controls were also evident by the lack of patient care protocols and staff training for the patient population cared for in this case. The root cause analysis revealed that the staff was not aware of the many risk factors of the obese patient undergoing this particular procedure. Although some of the staff had attended an in-service training session on the new procedure, a patient care protocol had not been developed to standardize the care practices and adequately prepare the health care team for the risks, care needs, and appropriate interventions for this patient population.

A risk factor of significance in this case is the anatomy of obese patients undergoing this surgery. Often their anatomy puts them at risk for a compromised airway, particularly when they are receiving narcotics that can also suppress respirations.

Lack of follow-up for a critical operation was shown through the failed oversight of the physician's behavior and his medical practice. Informally, two internists involved with the case expressed their unhappiness that the surgeon left town without ensuring adequate coverage the morning after elective surgery was performed on his patient.

The system *did* provide a standard that would ensure efficient and effective coverage for physicians who must leave town. The surgeon, however, did not follow the standard. When the surgeon's case underwent the peer review process through the medical staff, the surgeon's peers deemed the actions and treatment as "appropriate," and had no recommendations or sanctions. Therefore the system did not use its authority to insist on effective standards and did not implement proper actions for following up on deviant behavior.

CONCLUSIONS

This study of one error-event suggests that health care organizations must go beyond the root cause analysis approach of problem solving to include a whole-systems approach. The philosophy that errors occur because of the failures of practitioners must be reframed as one that views practitioners as valued members who create safety by overcoming hazards and providing safe environments. In this reframing, patient care errors are viewed primarily as a result of practitioners becoming overwhelmed by unsafe conditions rather than the fault of single individuals who fail. This view, in contrast to a constricted expectation of individual responsibility, promotes a whole-systems thinking approach that examines the systems, team dynamics, individuals, and collective norms, beliefs, and behaviors in the context of an error-event.

The TERCAP data collection instrument was pivotal in identifying individual and system contributors to error. Interviews added much additional information related to the team dynamics within the organizational context that would most likely not be available from a retrospective review of a practitioner's documentation of an event. Creating more reliable health care organizations requires that the organizational members, nurses, physicians, health care administrator leaders, and other employees possess an understanding of not only the chain of events that contribute to an error-event, but also of the individual, team, and collective norms and values that drive their behaviors in the organization. Further, a better understanding of these multiple contributors to error needs to evolve into a willingness to change fundamentally the way health care teams view their roles and the way leaders view the organization. Leaders have the responsibility of creating structures and managing organizations so that their practitioners and organizational members are supported and acknowledged for their role in patient safety, specifically practice breakdown prevention, intervention and mitigation.

References

Benner, P., Sheets, V., Uris, P., Malloch, K., Schwed, K., & Jamison, D. (2002). Individual, practice, and system causes of errors in nursing: A taxonomy. *Journal of Nursing Administration, 32*(10), 509-523.

Chassin, M. R., & Galvin, R. W. (1998). The urgent need to improve health care quality. Institute of Medicine National Roundtable on Health Care Quality. *Journal of the American Medical Association, 280*(11), 1000-1005.

National Council of State Boards of Nursing (NCSBN). (1995). *Delegation concepts and decision-making process National Council position paper.* Available online (with password) at www.ncsbn.org/public/regulation/delegation_documents_ delegati.htm. Accessed November 1, 2008.

Schwaninger, M. (2000). Managing complexity—The path toward intelligent organizations. *Systemic Practice and Action Research, 13*(2), 207-241.

Scott, K. (2004). *Errors and failures in complex health-care systems: Individual, team, system and cultural contributors.* Unpublished doctoral dissertation, Union Institute & University, Cincinnati.

Speelman, J. (2001). JCAHO Summary of the Sentinel Events Standard Requirements. *HealthBeat, 1*(1), 1-7.

INDEX

A

Access-related concerns, 25
Accuracy, 48
Activities (visible *vs.* invisible), 121
Adequate monitoring failure case
 case study, 162–169
 TERCAP analysis of, 165
Administration (medications),
 30–46
 case studies for
  chemotherapy protocol case,
   34–37
  groupthink error case, 37–39
  right medication-wrong route
   cases, 39–42
  TERCAP analyses of, 34,
   35–37, 38, 42–45
 fundamental perspectives of, 30,
  44–45
 multifactorial process roles in
  adverse effects, 30–31
  descriptions of, 30
  distractions, 31–32
  errors (latent *vs.* frontline), 31
  knowledge-base concerns, 31
  maximum disclosure, 32
  misinterpretation, 32–33
  NCSBN, 33
  outcomes, 32
  resource checks, 32, 33
  staffing concerns, 31–32
  state boards of nursing, 33–34
  systems design, 30–31.
   See also Systems design
   concerns.
  TERCAP frameworks, 33–34
Adverse effects, 30–31
Advocacy and responsibility,
 138–149
 attentiveness and surveillance
  concerns for.
   See also Attentiveness and
   surveillance.
 ANA Code of Ethics, 66–67
 lack of attentiveness, 65–66
 case study for
  misplaced affection-professional
   responsibility case,
   145–149
  TERCAP analysis of, 147–149
 diagnostic discernment and, 94
 interpersonal skills and, 141–142
 nurse-patient advocacy, 139–141
  centrality of, 139
  phronesis and, 140–141
  provider notification and, 139
  responsibility-specific concerns,
   139–141
 patient autonomy and, 142
 problem engagement and,
  141–142

Advocacy and responsibility
 (*Continued*)
 professional boundaries and,
  142–145
  crossing of, 144
  holistic approaches, 143
  professional behavior
   continuum, 143–144,
   143*f*
  violations of, 144–145
  zone of helpfulness, 143, 143*f*
Agency for Healthcare Research and
 Quality. *See* AHRQ (Agency
 for Healthcare Research and
 Quality).
Age-related hazards, 122–123
Aggressive behavior concerns,
 128–129
AHRQ (Agency for Healthcare
 Research and Quality), 162
ANA (American Nurses Association)
 Code of Ethics, 66–67
Assessment and data documentation,
 47–57
 case study for, 50–55
  late and later documentation
   case, 50–55
  TERCAP analysis of, 53–56
 current practices for, 47–48
 fundamental perspectives of,
  47–48, 56–57
  accuracy-related concerns, 48
  critical pathways charting,
   47–48
  exceptions, 47–48
  formats, 47–48
  outcome-based charting,
   47–48
  PIE charting, 47–48
  POMR charting, 47–48
  SOAP charting, 47–48
  teamwork, 47
  timeliness concerns, 48
 future perspectives of, 48–49
  documentation-care
   percentages, 49
  electronic systems, 48–49
  outcomes, 49
  standards, 48
  systems design, 48
  workflow, 48
 goals of, 47
 importance of, 48, 49
 NANDA and, 48
 NIC and, 48
 NOC and, 48
 principles of, 49
Attentiveness and surveillance,
 58–75
 case studies for
  attentiveness-surveillance
   breakdown case, 68–70

Attentiveness and surveillance
 (*Continued*)
  performance cross-monitoring
   case, 70–73
  TERCAP analyses of, 60*t*, 70,
   72–73
 challenges of, 66–67
 critical thinking and, 58
 definitions of, 60, 60*t*
 depersonalization and, 63
 diagnostic discernment and,
  78–79. *See also* Diagnostic
  discernment.
 disenburdening and, 58–59
 efficiency concerns for, 59
 engagement skills and, 63
 ethical *vs.* legal concerns of, 67
 failure to rescue, 61
 fatigue and sleep deprivation and,
  59
 formalism limitations and,
  63–64
 fundamental perspectives of, 58,
  73–74
 goals of, 58
 leadership and, 60
 morality-related concerns, 64–65
 overlapping practice and, 63
 professionalism and, 64–66
  ANA Code of Ethics, 66–67
  lack of attentiveness, 65–66
 recognition practices and, 63
 recommendations for, 68
 short-cut impacts, 59–60
 staffing and, 58, 59, 60–61
 systems design and, 58–59, 60,
  61–62. *See also* Systems
  design concerns.
 technology and, 62–63
 vigilance and, 59
 work overload concerns, 59–60
Attentiveness-surveillance
 breakdown case
 case study of, 68–70
 TERCAP analysis of, 70
Audit-related concerns, 109
Authorized provider orders
 interpretation, 130–137
 case study for
  TERCAP analysis of, 132*t*,
   134–135
 fundamental perspectives of,
  135–136
 misinterpretation sources,
  130–131
 safety systems design, 131–132.
  See also Systems design
  concerns.
  computerized documentation,
   131–132
  CPOE systems, 131–132
  flaws in, 132

171